CONTENTS

PREFACE

Developments in biomedical research, the practice of medicine, and the delivery of health care in the last thirty years have been dubbed by some a revolution. A direct effect of the biomedical revolution has been to raise for the health care practitioner, the patient, and society at large difficult and complex moral dilemmas with public policy implications.

Since the mid-1960s and throughout the 1970s, writers and practitioners in medicine, nursing, law, theology, philosophy, sociology, and some of the humanities, as well as shapers of public policy, have been grappling with the moral impact of the biomedical revolution. As "revolutionary" biomedical developments became standard medical practice, the general public heard ever more frequently about innovations and the questions they were creating. Public policy deliberation drew in foundations, citizens' committees, religious institutions, and other groups; the biomedical developments and the moral issues they had created were no longer the purview of specialists. In fact, many of the specialists who had lived longest with these issues called for deliberate efforts to broaden the discussion to include the informed general public.

Among those who called for an intentional effort to provide the general public with reliable information so that citizens could make their own informed decisions were some individuals active in the Society for Health and Human Values, a professional society of medical educators and others engaged since the mid-1960s in exploring the human values dimension of contemporary medical education. It has received support from United Ministries in Education (UME) from its inception. To respond to the growing need for inclusive public education and participation in the moral and public policy questions raised by the biomedical revolution, the Health and Human Values Program was established as a UME activity through a grant from the United Presbyterian Church, USA. I was made director of the Program at its inception in 1980.

It was first thought that a previous manuscript would be made ready for publication. However, readers found serious faults with its perspective. That experience, in addition to having observed similar attempts by other individual writers and organizations, convinced me that an attempt at a broad introductory book for a general audience would have to keep in balance a variety of perspectives. To achieve that goal, I asked two persons to join as co-contributors to this book: John Burnside, M.D., Professor of Internal Medicine and Associate Dean at the Hershey Medical Center of Pennsylvania State University, who, as Robert Wood Johnson Public Policy fellow for 1980, spent six months in a representative's office and six months in a senator's office working on health care legislation; and Tom Beauchamp, Ph.D., Professor of Philosophy and Senior Research Scholar at The Kennedy Institute of Ethics, Georgetown University, who is a prolific writer in the area of applied ethics, especially regarding issues with significant clinical practice and public policy implications.

The style we developed for writing the book called for me to construct all first drafts while Dr. Burnside was to have primary responsibility for the cases and all scientific and medical discussions. Dr. Beauchamp was responsible for the initial outline, annotated bibliography and selected readings and subsequently managed the completion of the final draft with other contributors. All collaborated in the total manuscript. We also asked Wendell Shackelford, Ph.D., a writer and communications consultant for various publications, to assist us with all revisions and with the book's design. Our goals would be enhanced, we realized, by the contributions of Joanne Trautmann, Ph.D., specialist in literature and medicine and Professor of Humanities and English at Hershey Medical Center. She selected the epigrams used in each chapter and allowed us to use some of her annotations for literary items in the bibliographies.

I would like to thank Mrs. Edna Boulden, who did most of the typing of all the drafts, and Miss Adaline Wentz, who always willingly and competently helped when needed; and the Advisory Team which made the Program possible in many ways—Ronald W. McNeur, Verlyn L. Barker, A. Myrvin DeLapp, and John W. Burnside, M.D.

This book, then, represents a collaborative effort. Such collaborations have pitfalls, and no doubt this book fell into some. But what has been achieved, we collectively believe, is a brief, introductory book for a general audience that examines complex issues from a variety of perspectives. It can also be a bridge for the reader's further exploration of the questions raised. We encourage the reader to *live with* these questions as they emerge and re-emerge in our lives as health care practitioners, patients, and citizens.

The issues explored here are complex, but not beyond our grasp. Some of them may be insolvable in any final sense, but at least a working consensus must be found for the sake of establishing the practices and laws and articulating the values by which we live. Throughout the 1980s and into the foreseeable future, they will become more vital, specific, and commonplace. This book is presented to the reader in the hope that he or she will be better prepared to cope in an era of values transition and to act as an informed participant in the choices we all face in the coming years.

—Frank M. Harron

INTRODUCTION

The questions addressed in this book are irresistible, and they are becoming increasingly familiar. Science delivers the power to alter reality, and we become concerned ethically about the "rightness" of intervention. When medical science offers new options in the realm of health, the quality of life, and death, no thoughtful person can remain detached from the ensuing debate.

Bioethical issues are receiving unprecedented coverage in both public and professional media, but awareness comes to us in fragments, heightening our interest and concern without really helping us to clarify our thoughts. Whether we are ready or not, we have new decisions to make. Developments in medicine and health care in the last thirty years have amounted to what some have called a biomedical revolution. In the past, the physician and other health care professionals have stood by in relative helplessness in the face of many diseases; now the health care professions manage a technological arsenal. For the treatment of many illnesses and injuries new options are available, which, even when they cannot produce recovery, may greatly affect the circumstances of life and death.

Now we have machines that can perform certain natural and necessary functions of the body. Organ transplantation has become almost commonplace. A woman's egg can be fertilized in a laboratory dish and be implanted in her womb, where it will develop into a new human being. Scientists are beginning to manipulate genetic materials in prescriptive ways. A list of examples could go on and on, each of which would imply the challenge to make choices among new alternatives. Patients, physicians, nurses, legislators, and, in fact, all citizens are discovering that choosing among medical aternatives is not exclusively a *medical* decision. Furthermore, the decisions can be very difficult when they involve a conflict among fundamental human values. When we have realized what *can* be done, we often must ask what *ought* to be done. When death seems near, ought a person be kept on a respirator? As genetic engineering increases our capacity to alter life, ought we seek to create a "better" human being? Advances in reproductive biology offer new opportunities to decide what human characteristics we select or do not select for increased or decreased frequency in future generations. Is it right to use these opportunities? For answers, we must probe beyond medicine and into the realm of morality.

Before we can say more about how these decisions involve moral choices, we wish to stress that we are not talking about a set of "moralistic" concerns. The word "moralistic" refers to concern with narrow interests, with conventional and even provincial moral attitudes. Those who are moralistic frequently are interested in upholding moral principles that dictate clear-cut right and wrong options. Instead, the moral choices we will discuss in this book are choices between at least two compelling alternatives, each of which can be justified by reference to serious, quite legitimate moral premises.

These kinds of choices are often made in the context of *dilemmas*. By definition, dilemmas present difficult choices precisely because there *are* at least two morally compelling alternatives. Since many of these choices are new, and since old choices such as abortion or euthanasia have taken on a new urgency, there is less than a clear working consensus about these matters of "right and wrong." It is not that all the "good" people who have all the "right" answers must hold out against all the "bad" people with all the "wrong" answers. The fact of the matter is that serious and responsible persons hold a diversity of views, even contradictory ones, and they can present valid moral defenses of the positions they hold.

We are living in an era of pluralism. Because ours is a fairly open society, debate can take place in the public forum. Churches promulgate positions; courts write precedent-setting opinions; special-interest groups educate and lobby; and professional societies and their journals take up issues of ethics and public policy. Moreover, academic professionals apply their disciplines to contemporary problems; states pass new laws; and the federal government searches for policies and guidelines. The public debate has seemed so urgent of late because this is a time of rapid and important transitions in personal and social values. Profound technological innovation always presents moral dilemmas and shakes our certainty about established values. Responsible, thoughtful persons sense the ground shifting, and feel anxious. They seek ways to cope with the anxiety, to influence the present and the future through policy. While the choices presented to us are the result of medical science, the decisions to be made transcend science.

We assume that you are reading this book because *you* are interested in vital choices as they arise in personal experience and, indeed, as they emerge in the processes of public deliberation. Our purpose is to present information and ideas that will aid in this deliberation, as it is the means by which a free and open society reaches a working consensus in law and policy.

Who shall decide, when doctors disagree,
And soundest casuists doubt, like you and me?

—Alexander Pope,
Moral Essays

FORMAT OF THE BOOK

Each chapter in this book contains actual case studies in medical practice and decision-making. The cases are intended to shed light on special issues within the chapter. Where it is appropriate, we will stop to present questions that may help you to focus on the essential concepts of the topic under discussion. We hope that you will think carefully about these questions at the point they are asked. When you reach the end of a chapter, we suggest that you return to the case study and the questions in order to ascertain any changes in your thinking and to reexamine the foundations of your decisions. Finally, chapter by chapter, we suggest that you identify those questions that continue to bother you.

The main portion of each chapter provides background discussion of key medical, moral, legal, and public policy factors that are important for understanding the issues. Where possible, we have provided charts, tables, and figures to summarize information or to highlight important points. Literary epigrams are included in order to emphasize that the problems discussed in this book are genuine and deep human concerns, not merely dispassionate "issues" unrelated to life and feeling. Shaw, Ibsen, Dickinson, Porter, Auden, and other poets, novelists, and playwrights remind us that our underlying concerns are not new and that art can enhance strikingly our understanding of health and human value questions.

After leading you through an analytical survey of the key issues in each chapter, we supply a group of selected readings by other authors. These readings take up some issues in more detail and usually argue various points of view on these issues. The readings are excerpts from the works of leading commentators in theology, law, philosophy, medicine, public health, and other relevant disciplines. Some of the excerpts are rigorous explorations of a particular point. Do not feel that you must read each excerpt as it arises; it is a legitimate shortcut to skip past a particular reading and perhaps return to it later. We believe that in the aggregate these readings will give you an accurate idea of the kinds of thinking that have been applied to problems of making moral choices in recent years and that they will increase your capacity to analyze problems in greater depth and detail.

The annotated bibliography at the end of each chapter offers some suggestions for still further exploration. We list books and articles usually available in most community or college libraries and comment on the significance of each. Two outside resources deserve special mention here: *The Encyclopedia of Bioethics*, edited by Warren T. Reich (New York: The Free Press, 1978), is an excellent general resource to which we will refer you more specifically in the annotated bibliography for each chapter; *Literature and Medicine: An Annotated Bibliography*, by Joanne Trautmann and Carol Pollard (Pittsburgh: University of Pittsburgh Press, 1982), selects and comments on hundreds of sources from literature, ancient to modern. Finally, we have included references to a few good audio/visual resources that deal with our topics.

Every book has to be selective. The topics that we have selected for discussion are intended to represent the *kinds* of choices confronting us today. We have not been able to include all areas of concern—for example, the moral and legal questions raised by developments in psychosurgery or behavior control. Some of the technologies that we do discuss still are relatively rare. So far, they have affected firsthand only a very small number of people. Early deliberation can contribute to responsible use of emerging technologies, and also can enable you, the reader, to cope with the impact of new technologies as they make their way into standard medical practice and health care.

Early impressions, in ethics or elsewhere, come to us in largely undifferentiated globs. Reason and analysis break them up and sort them out so that we can know what it really is that we are talking about.

—Daniel Maguire, *The Moral Choice*[1]

In consideration of any given issue, we will not presume to recommend any particular answer to questions of right and wrong. Instead, our purpose is to expose you to all major positions and arguments so that you may enlighten yourself through personal deliberation. Whether you are a doctor or a patient, a clergyperson, attorney, or interested layperson, a student

1. Daniel Maguire, *The Moral Choice* (Minneapolis: Winston Press, 1978), p. 262.

or a practicing professional, a lawmaker or a citizen who seeks to influence public policy, the issues in this book surely will touch your life directly. Public policy and moral choice both begin with discussion of coherent beliefs among individuals, and this process begins with orderly analysis of the issues.

1

MAKING MORAL DECISIONS

SIXTY-SEVEN-YEAR-OLD JOSEPH SAIKEWICZ HAD LIVED IN STATE INSTITUTIONS FOR OVER forty years. His mental age was approximately two years and eight months. He could communicate only by gestures and grunts. He was generally unresponsive to the people and things around him, was unaware of dangers, and became disoriented when removed from familiar places.

Surprisingly, Joseph's health was fairly good until April 1976, when he was diagnosed as having acute myelo-monocytic leukemia. This disease is inevitably fatal. In approximately thirty to fifty percent of cases, chemotherapy can bring about a temporary remission of symptoms, lasting between two and thirteen months. Results are even less hopeful for patients over sixty. Chemotherapy itself often has serious side effects, including anemia, nausea, vomiting, and infections.

At the petition of the Belchertown State School, where Saikewicz lived, the probate court appointed a guardian *ad litem* with authority to make necessary decisions concerning Joseph's care and treatment. (A guardian *ad litem* is appointed by a court to represent an incompetent person in a particular lawsuit.) The guardian noted that Joseph's illness was incurable and that therapy would create pain that Saikewicz would not be able to understand. The guardian argued that "not treating Mr. Saikewicz would be in his best interests."

On July 9, 1976, the Supreme Judicial Court of Massachusetts upheld the decision for Saikewicz *not* to receive standard medical treatment. Joseph Saikewicz died on September 4, 1976, of bronchial pneumonia.[1]

Before reading ahead, consider these questions.

1. Should Joseph Saikewicz have received standard medical treatment *regardless* of the consequences?
2. Is there a near-absolute duty that life-saving standard medical treatment should be administered *regardless* of the consequences?

1. *Superintendent of Belchertown State School* v. *Saikewicz*, 373 Mass. 728, 370 N.E.2d 417 (1977).

3. Did the consequences identified—namely, prolonged and incomprehensible suffering—justify withholding treatment from Saikewicz?
4. When a *patient* is incapable of making decisions, does *society* have the right to intervene and make a proxy decision for the incompetent person?
5. If *anyone* has the right to make a decision for a patient like Saikewicz, then *who,* exactly, should weigh the alternatives and make the decision?
6. Should such decisions always be left to the courts? Is that practical?
7. When such cases reach the courts, what are the relevant constitutional principles or general concepts concerning the rights of persons that seem applicable?

Do try to provide answers, even tentative ones, before reading further. It might be helpful to write down your initial answers so that you can reexamine them later.

The story of Joseph Saikewicz received a great deal of publicity. Its moral implications elicited comments from ethicists. Because the case went to court, the legal and public policy ramifications of it were widely discussed. The commentators who wrote about the case in newspapers, professional journals, and books examined it from many angles. Among the key points were these:

- Very often, modern medical techniques can provide a "partial victory" which may seem inhumane to some. It may be cruel to delay the death of some patients whose illnesses are hopeless and whose treatment would be very painful.
- Health care professionals face a dilemma: the fundamental precept of the profession is to save life, yet their personal, humanitarian instincts may cause them to question whether an all-out life-saving effort is morally defensible.
- The Saikewicz case presents an ethical problem not faced this keenly by previous generations: how do we decide who has the right to make life-and-death decisions for persons who are incapable of deciding for themselves?

One ethicist, Paul Ramsey, has argued that in the case of Joseph Saikewicz, and in similar cases, "the ethical rule of practice should be the treatment of incompetents always in the way normal patients would be treated."[2] He pointed out that the *average* person with this particular form of leukemia would seek the standard medical treatment—chemotherapy—in spite of the known side effects. Because of this, he concluded that the doctors, Belchertown State School, and the courts were obligated to make sure that Saikewicz received the same treatment the average person would accept. In the Saikewicz case, he accused the court of

---

2. Paul Ramsey, *Ethics at the Edges of Life* (New Haven: Yale University Press, 1978), p. 317.

"court-supervised involuntary euthanasia." He used the classic "slippery slope" argument, which reasons that when we allow one exception to a rule, we begin a downward slide, a dilution of the moral rule itself. Ramsey argued that the outcome of the Saikewicz case could open the door for doctors, the institutions of society, and the legal system to abandon their traditional roles in striving to save lives and protect rights of individuals.

The decision of the Supreme Judicial Court of Massachusetts affirmed that incompetent persons have the same right to refuse treatment as the average person has. However, in this case, since the wishes of the patient were unknown and unknowable, someone else had to make the decision for the patient. In the eyes of the court, doctors were not in a good position to make such decisions. The court said, "Such questions of life and death seem to us to require the process of detached but passionate investigation and decision that forms the ideal on which the judicial branch of the government was created. Achieving this ideal is our responsibility and that of the lower court, and is not to be entrusted to any other group purporting to represent the 'morality and conscience of our society,' no matter how highly motivated or impressively constituted."[3]

Imagine that you are a doctor faced with such a patient. Should you make the decision about his or her treatment, or should you go to court for instructions? How do you justify your answer to this question? Now think of yourself as the *patient*. Any one of us could be rendered incompetent, by a massive stroke, for example, and then contract a life-threatening illness. If this happened to you, who do you think should make the decisions about your treatment? your spouse? doctor? the courts?

The fact that these cases now are being decided individually in court, entailing much time and deliberation, demonstrates that our society as a whole is unprepared to deal with these moral and legal questions by means of well-established policy and consensus. We are still appraising our options. These special cases challenge previously accepted values about life, death, personhood, rights, the goals of medicine, and the responsibility of law.

MORAL REASONING COMBINES SEVERAL ELEMENTS

Throughout this book we will refer to certain concepts that facilitate what we shall call "moral reasoning." It will be helpful to identify some of these concepts here at the outset. Consider the following as working, but very elementary, descriptions of these concepts and terms.

3. Quoted in "Judges at the Bedside: The Case of Joseph Saikewicz," by George Annas, *Medicolegal News* 6 (Spring 1978): 11–12.

Moral reasoning includes the processes of analyzing, weighing, justifying, choosing, and evaluating competing reasons for an action.

Analyzing is breaking up the overall structure of a problem in a particular case into its leading alternatives.

Weighing means assessing the strengths and weaknesses of alternatives by balancing them against one another.

Justifying is done by providing a compelling and sufficient moral reason that appeals to an established moral principle, such as "Always tell the truth."

Choosing involves selecting one or more of the available alternatives, preferably on the basis of a position that can be and has been shown to be justified.

Evaluating includes reexamining the choices and their justifications, identifying unanswered questions, and relating decisions about one particular case to similar cases.

Moral reasoning stands in contrast to "intuitionism" and "casuistry." Intuitionism assumes that people with good character and educated minds intuitively know what is right and what is wrong. Casuistry, on the other hand, assumes that there is a specific, established rule for every situation. *Moral reasoning* assumes only that rules, principles, and concepts must be pursued in an orderly way to be useful in finding answers to new questions. An advantage of such a framework is that it opens a channel for concerned, informed persons to communicate diverse, and even contradictory, conclusions. (Moral dilemmas, by definition, are dilemmas because there are at least two compelling, defensible alternatives.) However, we do not mean to imply that moral reasoning is a step-by-step process which, if followed sequentially, produces "correct" answers automatically. By outlining and describing the elements that go into making moral choices, especially a choice in the context of a moral dilemma, we are making explicit the ways people generally deliberate and make a decision. These elements are a means of making one's position clear; they also increase the possibility for an open, democratic society, which is morally pluralistic, to debate and make informed public policy.

Now let us apply the elements that enter into moral reasoning, at least briefly, to the case of Joseph Saikewicz. *Analyzing* helps us to identify the major alternative courses of action in the case. We know that standard medical treatment for most patients suffering from this kind of leukemia is chemotherapy; that most patients accept this treatment; that if a competent person refuses treatment, the wish generally will be honored; and that Saikewicz was incompetent to make a decision for himself. Considering all these factors, the guardian *ad litem* argued that the best interests of Saikewicz would be served by withholding treatment. The two clear alternatives that form the nub of the dilemma in this case were to administer chemotherapy to the patient or to withhold it entirely.

The next job in moral reasoning is *weighing* the alternatives. Supporting the treatment are the facts that chemotherapy is standard practice for the illness, that most patients choose to receive the treatment, and that the prolongation of life was possible. That Saikewicz was incompetent to decide may be considered incidental to the importance of honoring his rights to receive every life-saving (or life-prolonging) treatment known to medicine. On the other hand, it may be argued that it is morally unjustifiable to force treatment on a patient who cannot comprehend the painful side effects. This position may seem more persuasive when we consider that even under the best circumstances chemotherapy in this case would prolong life for only a very short time.

Justifying is the process through which one joins a good and sufficient moral reason—grounded in a moral principle, which in turn is part of a comprehensive ethical system or theory—to the alternatives at hand. Usually one chooses on the basis of what one believes to be justifiable. This means simply that we try to justify our choices by relating them to general moral rules. In a genuine dilemma, this process of justification may force us to decide for the first time which of two highly valued principles we will place above the other. In the Saikewicz case, the court gave highest priority to withholding standard treatment because of the consequences that would ensue—painful, forced treatment that Mr. Saikewicz would not understand. Not causing harm was thereby considered a more compelling reason than prolonging, for a short period of time, life. *Choosing* is the stage at which one of the alternatives must be selected. The court chose *not* to treat Joseph Saikewicz, but by no means was there unanimity among the commentators on this case.

The final stage in moral reasoning is *evaluating*, the process of looking back on a particular choice and its consequences and deciding whether the course of action was clearly justified in light of one's exposure to similar moral problems. Right now, for example, how do you feel about the moral reasoning that predominated in the court in the Joseph Saikewicz case? Can you explain why you respond as you do? Which alternative do you regard as more morally defensible—to treat or not to treat?

ETHICAL THEORY

Most Western moral concepts fall within two leading types of ethical systems or theories—*deontological* theories and *utilitarian* theories. The word "deontology" is based on the Greek "deon," which means *duty*.

Deontology also has been called formalism and, by some writers, absolutism. Utilitarianism, by contrast, is a form of teleology (from the Greek "telos," which means *end* or *consequence*).

Deontologists hold that there are certain rigid duties that always are in force, no matter what the consequences may be. For example, in the case of Joseph Saikewicz, you remember that Paul Ramsey argued that incompetent patients should *always* be treated in the same way normal patients are treated. Utilitarians take a rather different perspective, although they, too, often defend a system with rigid rules. But their rules are based on some calculation of the consequences of decisions or actions. Again referring to Saikewicz, we noted that the argument was made that the consequences—uncomprehended suffering with little likelihood of positive results—justified an exception, in the eyes of the court, to the standard rule to treat all persons equally.

We have been discussing deontology and utilitarianism as if they existed in a pure form. Although some persons do come close to being pure deontologists or utilitarians, it is more common to find others who rely on some mixture of the two kinds of ethical systems and heavily qualify their commitment to whatever moral theory they promote. Our "pure characterizations" are, therefore, more like polar extremes, but taking this view of the theories will promote our understanding of the *basic* commitments of each.

Our polar-extreme approach may also lead one to anticipate that an individual's moral choices in a given case must be determined by aligning with one of these two theories, deontologists always voting one way and utilitarians always voting the other. This is by no means the case. Respected thinkers from both schools have used their theories to justify euthanasia, for example, whereas other experts have used both kinds of arguments *against* euthanasia. These theories are analytical tools or approaches, not steadfast prescriptions with predetermined moral outcomes. They could each be applied to the Saikewicz case, for instance, with a range of outcomes.

What, then, is the value of these analytical tools, which at first glance seem so arbitrary? Specialists in moral philosophy and theology use them as rallying points. To be identified as a deontologist or utilitarian indicates one's primary orientation in moral deliberation. One of the chief practical benefits for the person who is not a specialist in moral philosophy or theology is that understanding the two leading moral orientations in Western philosophy and theology helps to make explicit what he or she believes and does implicitly. Not only specialists, but also thoughtful persons generally are aware that they are heirs of the values of their culture. These values have been shaped by moral concepts articulated by previous generations from both creditable sources of moral thought.

Of these two leading moral orientations, deontology probably can be considered the older, because one source of deontological duty is considered by some to be divine revelation. Others have attributed the source to natural law, which its advocates say can be known by human reason. Still other people have claimed that absolute moral duties are knowable by human reason and common sense. As examples of these duties that obligate us regardless of the consequences, we can mention telling the truth, keeping promises, regarding persons as inviolable and never as a means to other goals, treating others as you want to be treated, etc.

Some deontologists, most notably Immanuel Kant (1724–1804), have tried to establish one duty as superseding all others. Kant hoped to find a "categorical imperative," the one duty which could be regarded by everyone, everywhere, in all times and places as a universal law. That duty—most popularly formulated as "Treat others as ends in themselves rather than as means to your own ends"—would take precedence over all other alternative courses of action. Other deontologists hold that instead of one universal, absolute duty, several basic rules—justice, truthfulness, regard for others, etc.—share priority. When these basic duties seem to conflict with respect to a certain dilemma, they try to determine which of the duties weighs the most, and moral reasoning is involved in this determination. For example, when a terminally ill patient wants to refuse further medical treatment, a conflict arises between the physician's duty to preserve life and combat illness on the one hand and the patient's right to self-determination on the other hand. Deontologists have argued this issue both ways, depending on which duty they see as overriding.

Utilitarianism regards most highly that which deontologists say is relatively unimportant—the *consequences* of a course of action. A utilitarian could argue that to override the autonomous choice of a patient who wishes to refuse treatment eventually will produce negative consequences for the human rights now ensured in the Bill of Rights. Another utilitarian might argue that if physicians start to withhold their best efforts to save life, regardless of the *reasons* for withholding the effort, the eventual consequence will be the undermining of confidence in the medical community.

All human decisions and actions have consequences. As far as utilitarians are concerned, right decisions are those that result in consequences that are ultimately valued, such as friendship, knowledge, financial security, and artistic achievement. Wrong decisions and actions are those that bring consequences that are ultimately disvalued, such as mistrust, pain, ignorance, financial ruin, barbarism in public and civic life. In general, utilitarians extend their reasoning to claim that right decisions are those that bring the greatest good for the greatest number of people. Naturally, disagreement arises over which consequences should be most valued. Imagine, for example, how much disagreement would be possible if this general utilitarian principle were applied to the Saikewicz case.

THE RELEVANCE OF RIGHTS

Recent medical developments have made "rights" a crucial question. In debating issues of abortion, for example, we talk about the rights of the woman and the rights of the fetus. In discussing euthanasia, there is much discussion about the patient's right to self-determination and right to die. Patients' rights now are debated in many therapeutic and experimental situations in which there is concern over the right to treatment and the right to health care. Even rights of unborn generations are examined in questions raised by developments in applied genetics. In sum, rights permeate the discussion of moral choices created by modern medical developments.

Both *moral* rights and *legal* rights are at stake in these discussions. In liberal, democratic societies, the establishment of legal rights is a dynamic, evolutionary process, not a static one. The impetus for change or expansion of legal rights frequently begins as a claim to a moral right—moral rights being considered more stable and not subject to the fluctuations of the political process. It is natural, then, that in the public debate about rights of persons there is, although at times unwittingly, constant appeal to moral reasoning.

One of the highly valued principles of our culture is that which holds that individuals should have maximum freedom of choice and action within a protected context of rights for the safety and welfare of society as a whole. This principle is known as a *negative right,* or right of noninterference. The Supreme Court decision of 1973 in *Roe v. Wade* upheld a negative right—the right of a woman to noninterference in the private decision about childbearing, in this case a decision about abortion. It is interesting to note that many Americans oppose abortion for themselves and their families yet are even more opposed to any law that would *limit* the freedom of individuals to decide this matter for themselves.

Positive rights are claims on someone to *provide* something; for example, the claim that citizens have a right to adequate health care is a statement of a positive right. This right makes a claim on society's health care resources and on the wealth of fellow citizens to provide some degree of access to health care for everyone, regardless of an individual's ability to pay. These theories about rights do not always provide as much help as we might wish, however, as the Saikewicz case might be used to show. Were Saikewicz's rights violated? If so, were his positive or negative rights violated? Also, all rights may come into serious conflict, as in the case of physicians' rights to self-determination conflicting with society's establishment of a right to health care.

MAKING PUBLIC POLICY

Moral rights are sometimes converted to legal rights through processes that create public policy. The Saikewicz case became, through the court system, a precedent-setting case, and in that respect a "public policy." In our system of government, the key policymakers include the president, the Congress, state legislatures, courts at all levels, and special agencies established by the nation and the states. Seeking to influence the direction of public policy are lobbyists, activists from various organizations, ranging from unions to churches and foundations, and individual citizens. The interaction of these agencies and forces eventually establishes public policy. It is a process carried on by deliberation and persuasion, moral reasoning and debate—and finally a determinative political process.

Public policy as it is related to medicine and health care has received an extraordinary amount of attention in this society. One precipitating reason is that the costs of health care have risen at a rate faster than the rate of inflation. Even the wealthiest modern societies realize that they have limited resources and must make decisions about how these limited resources will be spent. There is an unusually active moral element in the debate because health care so clearly affects the health and welfare of people. In addition to the question of expense and allocation of resources, there is another reason for the fervor that attends public debate about health care, which is that medical science has enabled health care professionals to make very dramatic advances—as in organ transplantation, artificial life support, prenatal testing and screening, and even genetic engineering. These capabilities have come upon us before we are ready as a society to agree on the moral propriety of various courses of action. The debate is ongoing, but one thing seems decided: an informed, articulate citizenry capable of careful moral deliberation is our best hope for developing sound, equitable public policy.

The discussion in this chapter has demonstrated a few of the ways that medical developments are creating new moral dilemmas with important, and sometimes vital, public policy ramifications. By examining the story of

Joseph Saikewicz, we have explored one way modern medicine raises the question of the moral status of persons, in this case especially persons who are not capable of making their own decisions. We have also seen how health care professionals may be faced with the dilemma of providing treatment that may sustain life but also may bring prolonged and even increased suffering. Through applying the analytical tools of theologians and philosophers, we have examined how some persons resolve moral dilemmas in favor of maintaining fixed rules in spite of conseqeunces while other persons regard consequences as the primary criterion for making moral decisions. Finally, we have briefly explored the questions of *who* should make some of the choices created by these new moral dilemmas. Should it be the doctors, the courts, or the society, through more explicit laws and policies? Some of these same points will reemerge in subsequent chapters; additional questions will also be raised. The stage has been set for examining how medical developments are raising new sorts of choices for us. At key points throughout the discussion, you will be encouraged to make your own decisions.

SELECTED READINGS
The Teleological View[4]

The basic concept of utilitarian ethics is, as its name indicates, the idea of utility: an act is right if it is useful. As soon as this is said the question arises, Useful for what end? For unless we know the end to which something is to be judged as a means, we do not know how to decide whether it is useful or not.

The answer given by utilitarianism is that an act is right when it is useful in bringing about a *desirable* or *good* end, an end that has *intrinsic value*. . . . A preliminary account . . . must be given if we are to understand utilitarian ethics. By "intrinsic value" is meant the value something has as an end in itself, and not as a means to some further end. This may be explained as follows. There are certain things we value because of their consequences or effects, but we do not value them in themselves. Thus we think it is a good thing to go to the dentist because we want healthy teeth and we have reason to believe that the dentist is a person who can help bring about this end. But few people find visiting the dentist good in itself. In other words, the act of visiting the dentist is done not for its own sake but for the sake of something else. This something else may in turn be valued not as an end in itself but as a means to other ends. Eventually, however, we arrive at certain experiences or conditions of life that we want to have and enjoy just for their own sake. These are ends that we judge to be intrinsically good; they have for us intrinsic value. The experience of undergoing dental treatment, on the other hand, has only instrumental value for us. We consider it good only because we

4. Excerpts from Paul Taylor, *Principles of Ethics: An Introduction*, pp. 55–82. (© 1975 by Dickenson Publishing Co., Inc. Reprinted by permission of Wadsworth Publishing Co.; Belmont, Calif. 94002.)

think it is a means to some further end. If we did not value the end, the means would lose its value. Thus suppose we did not mind losing our teeth or having toothaches. We would not then think going to the dentist was worthwhile. So the value of some things is entirely *derivative.* They derive all their value from the value of something else. Other things—things that are sought for their own sake—have *nonderivative* value. Their value is not derived from the value of something else and hence is intrinsic to them. Derivative value, in short, is instrumental value; nonderivative value is intrinsic value. . . .

Now the basic principle of utilitarian ethics is that *the right depends on the good.* This means that we can know whether an act is morally right only by finding out what its consequences are and then determining the intrinsic goodness (or badness) of those consequences. The moral rightness of an act is not itself an intrinsic value. On the contrary, an act is right only when it is instrumentally good and its rightness consists in its instrumental goodness. Our next question is, What is the standard of intrinsic value by which utilitarians judge the goodness of the consequences of a right act? Classical utilitarians have proposed two different answers to this. Some, like Jeremy Bentham, have said "pleasure;" others, like John Stuart Mill, have said "happiness," and have added that happiness is not merely a sum total of pleasures. A third answer has been suggested by a twentieth century utilitarian, G. E. Moore (1873–1958), who has claimed that intrinsic goodness cannot be defined in terms of either pleasure or happiness, but is a unique and indefinable property of things. Thus we have three types of utilitarianism, categorized according to these three views of the end to which morally right conduct is a means. They are called "hedonistic utilitarianism" (from the Greek word *hedone,* meaning pleasure); "eudaimonistic utilitarianism" (from the Greek word *eudaimonia,* meaning happiness or well-being); and "ideal utilitarianism" or "agathistic utilitarianism" (from the Greek word *agathos,* meaning good). . . .

The fundamental norm of hedonistic utilitarianism may be stated thus: An act is right if it brings about pleasure (or prevents the bringing about of pain); an act is wrong if it brings about pain (or prevents the bringing about of pleasure). The fundamental norm of eudaimonistic utilitarianism may be stated in a corresponding way, merely by substituting "happiness" for "pleasure" and "unhappiness" for "pain." Similarly, ideal or agathistic utilitarianism may be formulated by substituting "intrinsic good" for "pleasure" and "intrinsic evil" for "pain." As soon as the norm of utilitarian ethics is stated in any of these ways, another question immediately arises: Pleasure or happiness or intrinsic good *for whom,* pain or unhappiness or intrinsic evil *for whom?*

Many alternative answers are possible. One can say, pleasure, happiness, or intrinsic good for the agent himself, that is, for the person doing the act. The resulting ethical system would then be a form of ethical egoism. . . . Another possible answer is, pleasure, happiness, or intrinsic good for the agent's family and friends, or for the members of his class or caste, his tribe or nation, his race, religion, or sex. This would yield an ethical system in which the interests of some people are understood to have a greater claim to fulfillment than the interests of others. Still another possibility is, pleasure, happiness, or intrinsic good for everyone *but* the agent. This answer would entail an ethics of pure altruism or brotherly love, in which the moral ideal for each agent is to devote himself to the welfare of others at whatever cost to his own interests. Finally, the answer to our question which utilitarians give is, *everyone's* pleasure, happiness, or intrinsic good.

According to utilitarianism, whether it be hedonistic, eudaimonistic, or agathistic, the standard of value for judging the consequences of actions must be completely impartial and universal in its application. In calculating the positive or negative value of consequences, one person's pleasure (or happiness or intrinsic good) is to count exactly as much as another's. The agent's own interests are to be considered along with everyone else's, but no greater (and no lesser) weight is to be given to his interests than to those of any other individual. Between his own pleasure (happiness, intrinsic good) and that of someone else, the agent must be strictly impartial, never allowing himself to be prejudiced in his own favor or in favor of those whom he happens to like. All human beings, for the utilitarian, have an equal right to the fulfillment of their interests. . . .

To find out what one morally ought to do in any situation of choice, utilitarianism prescribes the following decision-making procedure. First we specify all the alternatives that comprise the possible courses of action open to our choice. We then calculate to the best of our ability the probable consequences that would ensue if we were to choose each alternative. In this calculation we ask ourselves, How much pleasure (or happiness) and how much pain (or unhappiness) will result in my own life and in the lives of all people who will be affected by my doing this act? When we have done this for all the alternatives open to us, we then compare those consequences in order to find out which one leads to a greater amount of pleasure (or happiness) and a smaller amount of pain (or unhappiness) than any other alternative. The act that in this way is found to *maximize intrinsic value and minimize intrinsic disvalue* is the act we morally ought to do. To do any other act in the given situation would be morally wrong.

In the practical affairs of everyday life, of course, we cannot stop and make such detailed calculation every time we have alternative courses of action open to us. Indeed, if we were to do this we might cause more unhappiness or less happiness to be brought about in the world than if we were to make choices on the basis of habits we had developed from our past experience. Thus it would be wrong for us, according to the principle of utility, to try to make an accurate calculation each time. What we must do is to use our common sense and choose on the basis of similar situations in the past. After all, it does not take much thought to predict that murdering someone is going to produce more unhappiness in the world than respecting the person's life. We need not have committed a murder in the past to know this. We need only to use our reason and imagination to be able to make a reasonable prediction about what would happen if we were to do such an act.

It is important to realize that for the utilitarian no act is morally wrong in itself. Its wrongness depends entirely on its consequences. Take the act of murder, for instance. If the consequences of murdering a particular man in a particular set of circumstances (say, assassinating Hitler in 1935) were to bring about less unhappiness in the world than would be caused by the man himself were he to remain alive, it is not wrong to murder him. Indeed, it is our duty to do so, since the circumstances are such that our refraining from doing the act will result in more unhappiness (intrinsic disvalue) and less happiness (intrinsic value) than our doing it. This might at first appear to be a shocking and outrageous teaching. But the utilitarian would argue, What, after all, is wrong with the act of murder? Is it not that it causes so much pain and unhappiness both to the victim and to his kin, and prevents the victim from having the chance to enjoy his right to the pursuit of happiness?

The Deontological View[5]

Deontological theories deny what teleological theories affirm. They deny that the right, the obligatory, and the morally good are wholly, whether directly or indirectly, a function of what is nonmorally good or of what promotes the greatest balance of good over evil for self, one's society, or the world as a whole. They assert that there are other considerations that may make an action or rule right or obligatory besides the goodness or badness of its consequences—certain features of the act itself other than the *value* it brings into existence, for example, the fact that it keeps a promise, is just, or is commanded by God or by the state. Teleologists believe that there is one and only one basic or ultimate right-making characteristic, namely, the comparative value (nonmoral) of what is, probably will be, or is intended to be brought into being. Deontologists either deny that this characteristic is right-making at all or they insist that there are other basic or ultimate right-making characteristics as well. For them the principle of maximizing the balance of good over evil, no matter for whom, is either not a moral criterion or standard at all, or, at least, it is not the only basic or ultimate one. . . .

Deontological theories are also of different kinds, depending on the role they give to general rules. *Act-deontological theories* maintain that the basic judgments of obligation are all purely particular ones like "In this situation I should do so and so," and that general ones like "We ought always to keep our promises" are unavailable, useless, or at best derivative from particular judgments. Extreme act-deontologists maintain that we can and must see or somehow decide separately in each particular situation what is the right or obligatory thing to do, without appealing to any rules and also without looking to see what will promote the greatest balance of good over evil for oneself or the world. . . .

Rule-deontologists hold that the standard of right and wrong consists of one or more rules—either fairly concrete ones like "We ought always to tell the truth" or very abstract ones like Henry Sidgwick's Principle of Justice: "It cannot be right for A to treat B in a manner in which it would be wrong for B to treat A, merely on the ground that they are two different individuals, and without there being any difference between the natures of circumstances of the two which can be stated as a reasonable ground for difference of treatment."[a] Against the teleologists, they

---

5. Excerpts from William Frankena, *Ethics*, 2d ed., © 1973. Adapted by permission of Prentice-Hall, Inc., Englewood Cliffs, N.J.

a. Henry Sidgwick, *The Methods of Ethics*, 7th ed. (London: Macmillan and Co., Ltd., 1907), p. 380.

insist, of course, that these rules are valid independently of whether or not they promote the good. Against act-deontologists, they contend that these rules are basic, and are not derived by induction from particular cases. . . .

Usually rule-deontologists hold that the standard consists of a number of rather specific rules like those of telling the truth or keeping agreements, each one saying that we *always* ought to act in a certain way in a certain kind of situation. Here, the stock objection is that no rule can be framed which does not admit of exceptions (and excuses) and no set of rules can be framed which does not admit of conflicts between the rules. To this objection, one might say that an exception to a rule can only occur when it has to yield the right of way to another rule, and that the rules proposed may be ranked in a hierarchy so that they never can conflict or dispute the right of way. One might also say that the rules may have all the necessary exceptions built into them, so that, fully stated, they have no exceptions. Thus, for example, the case of the white lie, if we accept it, is an exception to the rule "We ought never to lie," but if we formulate the "exception" as part of the rule and say, "We ought not to lie, except for white lies," assuming that we have a way of telling when a lie is "white," then it is no longer an exception. It must be confessed, however, that no deontologist has presented us with a conflict-and-exception-free system of concrete rules about what we are actually to do. To this fact, the deontologist might retort, "That's the way things are. We can't be as satisfied with any other theory of obligation as with this one, but this one isn't perfect either. The moral life simply does present us with unsolvable dilemmas." But, of course, we need not agree without looking farther. . . .

A rule-deontologist can avoid the problem of possible conflict between basic principles if he can show that there is a single basic non-teleological principle that is adequate as a moral standard. One such monistic kind of rule deontology with a long and important history is the Divine Command theory, also known as theological voluntarism, which holds that the standard of right and wrong is the will or law of God. Proponents of this view sometimes hold that "right" and "wrong" *mean,* respectively, commanded and forbidden by God, but even if they do not define "right" and "wrong" in this way, they all hold that an action or kind of action is right or wrong if and only if and *because* it is commanded or forbidden by God, or, in other words, that what ultimately *makes* an action right or wrong is its being commanded or forbidden by God and nothing else.

One who holds such a view may believe that we ought to do what is for the greatest general good, that one ought to do what is for his own good, or that we ought to keep promises, tell the truth, etc. Then his working ethics will be like that of the utilitarian, ethical egoist, or pluralistic deontologist. In any case, however, he will insist that such conduct is right because and only because it is commanded by God. If he believes that God's law consists of a number of rules, e.g., the Ten Commandments of the Old Testament, then, of course, like the pluralistic rule-deontologist, he may still be faced with the problem of conflicts between them, unless God somehow instructs us how to resolve them. . . .

It is not easy to discuss the Divine Command theory of right and wrong in a way that will satisfy both believers and nonbelievers. The latter find the theory hard to take seriously and the former find it hard to think that, if God commands something, it may still be wrong. We must remember, however, that many religious thinkers have rejected the Divine Command theory, at least in its voluntaristic form.

ANNOTATED BIBLIOGRAPHY
Books and Articles

Beauchamp, Tom L. *Philosophical Ethics.* New York: McGraw-Hill, 1981. A comprehensive treatment of contemporary moral philosophy that uses a case-analysis approach in each chapter. The writing is exceptionally clear, and the book includes detailed bibliographies and brief selections from major classical and contemporary writers.

————and Childress, James F. *Principles of Biomedical Ethics.* New York: Oxford University Press, 1979. Chaps. 1 and 2. The most widely used systematic analysis of ethical theory and medicine. This book takes an entirely theory-based and principle-based approach to the subject (rather than a topical approach), but includes many perspectives.

MacIntyre, Alasdair. *A Short History of Ethics.* New York: Macmillan, 1966. A clearly written study of the leading periods and persons in the history of philosophical ethics. Very much written from MacIntyre's own distinct perspective.

Nielsen, Kai. "Problems of Ethics." In *Encyclopedia of Philosophy,* ed. Paul Edwards. New York: Macmillan and Free Press, 1967. Vol. 3, pp. 117–34. An analytical outline of the important problems in modern ethical theory; comprehensive yet brief.

Rachels, James. "Can Ethics Provide Answers?" *Hastings Center Report* 10 (June 1980): 32–40. A clearly written essay on the role of applied ethics in the resolution of moral problems in one of the leading journals in biomedical ethics.

U.S., National Commission for the Protection of Human Subjects of Biomedical and Behavioral Research. *The Belmont Report: Ethical Guidelines for the Protection of Human Subjects of Research.* DHEW Publication No. (OS) 78–0012. Washington, D.C.: Government Printing Office, 1978. A publication that exhibits moral theory at work in public policy. This commission issued the document in order to explain the principled framework it used to examine a wide variety of problems in research with human subjects. (See chapter 5 of this volume for some details of this commission's work.)

Anthologies

Gorovitz, Samuel, ed. *Mill: Utilitarianism, with Critical Essays.* New York: Bobbs-Merrill, 1971. A well-introduced and carefully organized volume that ranges beyond Mill's analysis to broader problems about utilitarianism.

Lyons, David, ed. *Rights.* Belmont, Calif.: Wadsworth Publishing Company, 1979. A collection of relatively technical but first-rate essays on the nature of rights-claims and the language of rights.

Taylor, Paul W., ed. *Problems of Moral Philosophy*, 3rd edition. Belmont, Calif.:
Dickenson Publishing Company, 1978. Chap. 1. For many years this carefully
introduced and edited volume has been among the most respected textbooks in
moral theory. The topics include the nature of morality, relativism, egoism,
classical moral theories, freedom and determinism, and fact-value problems.

Articles from the *Encyclopedia of Bioethics*

Ethics
   I. The Task of Ethics *John Ladd*
   II. Rules and Principles *Wm. David Solomon*
   III. Deontological Theories   *Kurt Baier*
   IV. Teleological Theories *Kurt Baier*
   V. Situation Ethics *Joseph Fletcher*
   VI. Utilitarianism *R. M. Hare*
   VII. Theological Ethics *Frederick S. Carney*
   VIII. Objectivism in Ethics *Bernard Gert*
   IX. Naturalism *Carl Wellman*
   X. Non-Descriptivism *R. M. Hare*
   XI. Moral Reasoning *Philippa Foot*
   XII. Relativism *Carl Wellman*
Rights
   I. Systematic Analysis *Joel Feinberg*
   II. Rights in Bioethics *Ruth Macklin*

Literature

Hejinian, John. *Extreme Remedies*. New York: St. Martin's Press, 1974. A first
novel by a doctor-writer. The world of modern medicine is described accurately
and entertainingly, in the way of all good novels. The expected characters are
present, including an idealistic intern and other doctors who are interested in
lots of money and important reputations. The central character is enmeshed in
the politics and moral dilemmas of modern medicine and health care.
Crane, Stephen. "The Monster." In *The Complete Short Stories and Sketches of
Stephen Crane*, ed. T. A. Gullason. Garden City: Doubleday and Co., 1963.
Written in the nineteenth century, this short story traces the consequences of a
doctor's life-saving act. A doctor's servant, Henry Johnson, is badly mutilated in
an accident while saving his master's son. Dr. Trescott successfully saves Johnson's life, although against the advice of a good friend, a judge: "He is purely
your creation. Nature has evidently given him up. He is dead. You are restoring
him to life. You are making him, and he will be a monster with no mind."

Audio/Visual

"Joan Robinson: One Woman's Story." 165-minute film or videotape. Sale or
rental, Time/Life Video, Eisenhower Drive, Paramus, N.J., 07652. A bold, startling record of Joan Robinson's battle against cancer in the modern medical
context. The *cinema verité* style lays bare the feelings, dilemmas, and issues for

all involved. Among the themes explored are the patient-physician relationship, right to refuse treatment, informed consent, and patient care for the terminally ill. The same documentary footage has been used by Time/Life to create six 30-minute programs that include commentaries from physicians, clergy, nurses, attorneys, and others.

2

THE VALUE AND RIGHTS OF HUMAN LIFE: ABORTION AND PRENATAL PROCEDURES

MELINDA ALLEN, 17, WAS THE OLDEST OF THREE DAUGHTERS. HER FATHER WAS A HIGHLY respected local businessman and her mother served on the school board. Dr. Stevens, the family physician, had provided care to all members of the Allen family from time to time over the years and knew them all well.

Melinda had become sexually active at age 16 and Dr. Stevens had given her a prescription for contraceptive pills. About a year later, Melinda appeared in his office, six weeks pregnant, asking him to arrange an abortion for her; she had never filled the prescription. Dr. Stevens said that he was being put in a very difficult position as Melinda had not confided in her parents and Dr. Stevens knew that both of them were vocal in their opposition to abortion. In fact, Dr. Stevens himself had a personal and professional reluctance to recommend abortions. Melinda stated clearly that she did not want the baby, that she had adequate funds of her own to pay for the abortion, and that she expected absolute confidentiality to be maintained. *Dr. Stevens felt that as a physician he had some responsibilities to the fetus and to Melinda's parents as well as to Melinda herself.* He anticipated that eventually Melinda's parents would find out about the abortion and that they would consider that their doctor had deceived or even betrayed them. Stevens dreaded that possibility.

The complications did not stop there. During his discussion with Melinda, Dr. Stevens learned that the father of the baby wanted to marry Melinda and that he very much wanted her to have the baby. Still, the law at this time was explicit: Melinda had the legal right to her abortion and to confidentiality in the matter. Neither the baby's father nor Melinda's parents had any rights under the law.

Dr. Stevens felt that he could not act in the situation without first coming to grips with his own feelings. Personally he felt that the appropriate thing to do was to encourage Melinda to discuss her situation with her boyfriend and her parents. He reasoned that after talking openly with them any decision that Melinda made would be a more responsible one and that he himself could no longer be accused of being deceptive. Stevens felt angry at Melinda, especially because he had foreseen the possibility of an unwanted pregnancy and had taken steps to try to prevent it from happening.

Melinda steadfastly refused to confer with her boyfriend or her parents. Stevens searched his mind for an acceptable, disinterested third party with whom Melinda might discuss her situation before reaching a final decision but he could find none. He considered making his assistance conditional on Melinda's speaking with her parents first, but he could not honestly justify that course either. He considered the possibility of refusing any assistance at all, given that the situation was not an emergency and that alternative centers were available in the community. Stevens concluded that for him abortion was not consistent with what he considered to be the proper goals of the practice of medicine. He gave Melinda the name of a trusted colleague in another town, a doctor whom he knew did not share his reservations about abortion.

Some Questions to Consider
1. Who ought to have the final say in this case regarding a decision to abort or not to abort Melinda's fetus? Her parents, her boyfriend, Dr. Stevens, Melinda, or society, through a law to protect the unborn fetus?
2. What reasons—moral or legal—can you give to justify your choice?
3. What is the status of the fetus implicit in your answers to these first two questions? Is it a human being, a potential human being, a subdividing fertilized egg, or of some other category you can describe?

A TAPESTRY OF ISSUES

Melinda's situation has been repeated hundreds of thousands of times in families all over the country. Even assuming that Melinda's parents remained unaware of her situation, there still were several people wrestling with intense feelings based on personal, moral, and legal concern. The stimulus behind all this intensity was the existence of a tiny fetus.

Our understanding of the dynamics of human reproductive biology represents fairly recent knowledge for humankind. Although medical science has documented the microscopic circumstances of conception and the cellular and embryonic stages leading to birth, people still tend to regard with wonder the very notion of the beginning of a new life. Through the ages we have reserved for this subject a high place in our folklore and mythology, in our philosophy and religion, in our technical and scientific probes into the remaining unknown. Few subjects carry with them more intensity of feeling, and adding to that intensity is our recently discovered ability to *intervene* in matters of genetics, conception, and fetal development.

The status of the fetus, the rights of the woman, and society's role in defining and prescribing those rights are the three areas most in need of careful analysis in this complex and emotional issue. Stated starkly, the contrary positions can be put this way:

- Conception is "the moment of humanization."

- In the biological development of a human being, there is no "moment" that delineates humanization. The point of the beginning of humanization has varied in many cultures and different times. Placing it at conception is a value judgment that is not self-evident to all.

- Just as society—through its moral precepts and laws—is obligated to protect the rights of all persons, so it is obligated to protect the rights of the developing human being from the "moment of conception" onward. Therefore, society is justified, indeed obligated, to intervene in order to protect the life of the fetus.

- With no moral consensus about when human life begins, the society—through its moral precepts and laws—must protect the privacy of the woman in making her own decision regarding her fetus.

Perhaps these simple summaries will provide a loose end with which to begin untangling the complex and emotional issues at stake: the status and rights of the fetus in comparison with the rights of the woman and the society's role in prescribing and protecting those rights.

Abortion is the best-known social controversy that raises profound moral issues in the lives of individual women and their families. Still, it is not the only issue which does so. Fetal research and laboratory experimentation with alternative procedures of human reproduction are two other biomedical procedures concerning which these issues arise. The intra-uterine contraceptive device, which expels a fertilized egg from the womb, is another example of a medical technology that raises new moral and legal questions. Developments such as genetic testing and prenatal diagnosis make the dilemmas sharper.

The following discussion begins with a medical procedure, namely *in vitro* fertilization, that raises few moral objections for most people. We then consider fetal research, which *does* raise qualms for many people about the status of the fetus. Next we consider the current moral impasse on abortion between those who believe conception is the "moment of humanization" and those who believe that no such "moment" exists but instead opt for the decision-making of the woman to supersede in such situations. We then examine how the current legal and public policy situation favors the right of the woman to a private decision without interference from others. Finally, we test the limits of your acceptance of the woman's private decision in cases where prenatal testing leads to an abortion decision for a "serious" reason (the fetus has Down's syndrome) or a "trivial" reason (a child of the opposite sex was wanted).

FERTILIZED EGGS AND FULL HUMAN STATUS

LOUISE JOY BROWN, A 5 LB., 12 OZ. BABY GIRL, WAS BORN AT 11:47 P.M. ON JULY 25, 1978. The doctor who delivered her described her as chubby and muscular. Louise's arrival was a remarkable and gratifying event for her parents, who previously had been unable to have children. Louise was important in another way, too: she was the first baby in history to be born of her mother, but conceived in a medical laboratory outside her mother's body. Louise Joy was conceived when her father's sperm and her mother's egg were united in a glass dish. The press called her the first test-tube baby.

Lesley Brown, Louise's mother, was unable to conceive children naturally because her fallopian tubes were blocked, absolutely preventing fertilization of an egg. According to some estimates, 2 percent of the women in child-bearing age are infertile because of this condition. For many women and their husbands, the inability to conceive produces deep self-doubt and anguish. The distress of women like Lesley Brown is what motivated Dr. Patrick Steptoe, a British gynecologist, to recruit the aid of Dr. Robert Edwards, a geneticist.

Together they carried out a bold experiment. They removed an egg from Mrs. Brown's ovary and fertilized it with her husband's sperm in a glass petri dish. Three days later, the doctors implanted the tiny mass of multiplying cells into Mrs. Brown's womb. From that point on, the pregnancy proceeded normally.

By the time Dr. Steptoe and Dr. Edwards were ready to carry out this procedure, they had engaged in many years of careful study and preparation. Even during this time they were attacked by some people who believed that they were "tampering with life," moving into realms in which they had no authority. Some religious groups, protesting that the doctors and scientists were destroying human life by destroying embryos, attacked the work as immoral.

Those who opposed the Steptoe-Edwards procedure did so on the basis of a concern for the life of the embryo. At the root of that concern is the argument that human life begins at the moment of conception and from that moment on is entitled to all rights usually given to human beings. Steptoe and Edwards openly admitted that when they were doing their laboratory work some fertilized eggs (up to several days old) were un-

Table 1 Some Major Normal Stages in Fetal Development

Time	Cardiovascular system	Nervous system	Other criterion
Some Hours	—	—	Intercourse followed by "capacitation"
0 Hours	—	—	Fertilization; 1 cell, often called *zygote*
About 22 hours	—	—	2 cell Possible recombination
About 44 hours	—	—	4 cell until day?
About 66 hours	—	—	8 cell Possible twinning
About 4 days	—	—	16 cell until day 14 *Morula* stage
About 6–7 days	—	—	Implantation—often called *blastocyst* stage
2 weeks	—	—	Name changed from zygote to *embryo*
3–4 weeks	Heart pumping	—	—
6 weeks	—	—	All organs present
7–8 weeks	—	Mouth or nose tickling-neck flexing	—
8 weeks	—	Readable brain electric activity	Name change from embryo to *fetus*. Length 3 cm.
9–10 weeks	—	Swallowing, squinting, local reflexes	—
10 weeks	—	Spontaneous movement	—
11 weeks	—	—	Thumb sucking
12 weeks	Fetal EKG via mother	—	Brain structure complete Length 10 cm.
13 weeks*	—	—	D&C contraindicated hereafter
12–16 weeks*	—	—	"Quickening." Length 18 cm. at 16 weeks
16–20 weeks*	Fetal heart heard	—	Length 25 cm. at 20 weeks
20 weeks*	—	—	Name change from abortus to premature infant
20–28 weeks*	—	—	10% survive
28 weeks*	—	—	Fetus said to be "viable" in some definitions
40 weeks*	—	—	Birth

*Calculated from the first day of the last menstrual period.

Source: Andre Hellegers, "Fetal Development," *Theological Studies* 31 (March 1970): 8.

avoidably destroyed. Some were disposed of because they appeared less likely to develop normally when implanted; others were destroyed in the process of placing them between glass plates for examination under a microscope. Steptoe and Edwards disclosed that in some cases the requirements of their research had resulted in their destroying embryos up to two weeks old.

Their critics accused them of murder. This accusation is one that you will recognize can result from certain deontological theories in ethics. Under the assumption made by those deontologists who believe conception is the beginning of human life, the duty to protect developing human life is absolute, and anything less is a violation of all that is sacred and unique about human life. For them, the fertilized, developing egg, regardless of the stage of development, is entitled to the full rights of protection granted to each and every human being. This position is a deontological principle of respect for (human) life, a principle utilitarians (and *many* deontologists) have usually not taken as overriding in the case of fetal life.

Dr. Robert Edwards answered the critics for himself and for Dr. Steptoe in a utilitarian language that rejects "absolutist" deontological theories:

Patrick knew, as I did, that there would always be some embryos that would not be replaced in their mothers. Instead they would have to be examined, they would have to be fixed and stained for microscopic examination, and as a result, their growth ended. Was it justifiable to use these blastocysts so that we could investigate early human growth? Did they have any rights? Society at large appears to allow them rights, not at fertilization, but later in pregnancy. The intra-uterine devices of conception that some women wear ensure that any cleaving embryos are expelled and lost naturally without anyone even being aware of them. Indeed, abortion laws remove the right to life from much older foetuses, including those with inherited defects at three to four months of gestation if their handicap is too big to be accepted by their parents. The embryos cleaving in our culture fluids were minute and immature without the vestige of an organ or even a tissue compared with those aborted under the law.

Of course, absolutists disagree. [The British frequently use "absolutist" for "deontologist."] They regard fertilization as a kind of holy event above the interference of man. The overwhelming consensus of society and its laws, as well as many observations in biology, do not sustain the absolutist point of view about fertilization as the essential step that instantly confers on the fertilized cell the full rights of the individual. As a matter of fact, life is highly organized in the egg before fertilization and an embryo can develop to advanced stages of growth by being stimulated artificially by that process called parthenogenesis. A single blastocyst is not the pinpoint of one life necessarily: it will on occasion divide to produce two, three, four or even five identical offspring, each capable of normal life. Fertilization is for me but one step on the long road to birth. And there are many other fundamental steps on the way.[1]

After having refuted to his satisfaction the contention that human life in its fullest sense begins at the moment of conception, and offering instead a gradualist's understanding of human involvement, Edwards turned directly to utilitarian arguments. He attempted to justify his and Dr. Steptoe's work in terms of the benefits for innumerable persons of the future scientific applications and therapeutic advances made possible by it:

These embryonic cells contain mysteries that can and must be solved—how they increase rapidly and then successively grow into different organs during early growth. And most exciting of all, they may possibly be used in treating many human disorders.

We need more knowledge of these very early stages if we are to discover how it is that illnesses such as German measles or drugs such as thalidomide interfere with normal development. Perhaps we can find some clues, however small, if we observe the growing sensitivity and susceptibility to such harmful agents of cells growing in the embryo in culture. Perhaps we shall be able to understand why other embryos succumb and become invasive to their own mother, threatening her by their massive, disordered challenge. Any knowledge along these lines, however meager, would be a help.

Will we be able to discover how these cells appear and develop so regularly? Will we be able to extract the stem cells of various organs from the embryo, the precious foundation cells of all the body's organs and then use them therapeutically? Will it ever be possible to use these cells to correct deficiencies in other human beings—to replace one deficient tissue with another that functions normally? For instance, will we be able to use the blood-forming cells of an embryo to re-colonize defective blood-forming tissue in an adult or child? And will these notions be met with pursed lips and frowning faces?

Perhaps the whole concept will fall to the ground and prove to be a mistaken one in medical treatment. I doubt it. So much is on our side—the very foundation cells have been and will be again in our cultures and we know they are capable of displaying the initial signs of tissue differentiation. These same embryonic cells may be offering us one further therapeutic advantage. They may one day be used without having to worry about graft rejection such as we all know is associated with kidney, heart and liver transplantations.

Perhaps this whole approach may seem heartless to those who feel the embryo is a human being who must be protected at all costs. I cannot share this opinion. If we can alleviate certain disorders in children or adults who are suffering greatly or who may be dying, then surely we must be allowed to use these cells, taken from an embryo while still only the size of a pinhead—stem cells collected and grown in cultures until they can be used to repair damage or defect.

To grow foetuses to later stages of growth when they take a recognizable human

1. Robert Edwards and Patrick Steptoe, *A Matter of Life*, pp. 96–97. Copyright © 1980 by Finestride Ltd. & Crownchime Ltd. By permission of William Morrow & Co.

shape and then extract their organs would be utterly wrong and is a repugnant concept; but to obtain cell colonies from minute embryos useful in medicine for the alleviation of certain human disorders—is that not a legitimate target to aim at? It is a target that may be reached, should be reached, if we can understand the priceless secrets of those embryonic cells growing in our cultures.

We know that our work is opening new horizons in human reproduction—indeed, it has already opened some. We are aware, too, that it introduces the possibility of genetic engineering or embryological engineering in one form or another, as feared by those [newspaper] correspondents ten years ago when we first began our work. Now that we have demonstrated that human conception can occur outside of the human body, many investigations can be done which were impossible before.[2]

To many persons, Dr. Edwards's suggestion seems plausible: it is not appropriate to describe an embryo as a human being when it is "still the size of a pinhead." Even more convincing for those who take this view is his argument that society benefits from such work, although some embryos are inevitably lost or destroyed. The woman who was unable to have children due to blocked fallopian tubes can now do so, and the advance of medical science is inestimable. The embryo is tiny, does not have any human features, and seems dispensable when the benefits to individuals and society are great. In short, the beneficial consequences to couples and to society's advancing knowledge of fetal development justified their work, even though embryos were lost, in the eyes of Steptoe and Edwards. Of course, one can imagine that many deontologists would resist such arguments. Moreover, what about destruction of fetuses at a *later* stage of development? Research and medical procedures in which embryos are lost in the first weeks of pregnancy (which can happen spontaneously, even without the mother's awareness) is one thing, some may feel, but the destruction of a fetus of up to twenty weeks gestational age may be unacceptable. Why?

FETAL RESEARCH

Before 1973, most research on fetuses in the United States was performed on those fetuses that were expelled by spontaneous abortions. When the Supreme Court legalized access to abortion in 1973, many more fetuses were available for research. Society clearly needed some guidelines to specify the conditions under which fetuses could be used in this way. The medical community in general has been persistent in claiming the value of fetal research. Researchers have pointed out, for example, that nonliving, spontaneously aborted fetuses were crucial for culturing the viruses that

2. Ibid., pp. 186–87.

led to the creation in the 1940s of a polio vaccine. Once society accepted the general idea that research might be done on fetuses at all, guidelines were nevertheless needed to govern such research activities.

In 1974, Public Law 93–348 established the National Commission for the Protection of Human Subjects of Biomedical and Behavioral Research, one of whose functions was to study issues in great detail and forward recommendations to Congress and appropriate agencies. On May 17, 1978 the commission published a summary of its recommendations concerning research on the fetus:

The Commission affirmed its belief that the fetus, as a human subject, should be treated with respect and dignity regardless of its life prospects. Because some information that is in the public interest and provides significant advances in health care can be attained only through the use of the human fetus as a research subject, the Commission recommended that research involving the human fetus should be conducted and supported under limited conditions and with careful ethical review.

The Commission recommended that therapeutic research involving the fetus may be permitted if it conforms to appropriate medical standards and has been approved by an Institutional Review Board. Nontherapeutic research directed towards the fetus *in utero* may be conducted if: (1) the knowledge to be gained is important and cannot be obtained by alternative means, (2) appropriate investigations on animals have been completed, (3) the research presents no more than minimal risk, and (4) the research has been approved by an Institutional Review Board; if such research is in anticipation of abortion and there are problems in applying these guidelines, it may be conducted if approved by a national ethical advisory body. Nontherapeutic research during abortion or directed at the nonviable fetus *ex utero*, must satisfy three additional guidelines: (1) the fetus must be less than 20 weeks gestational age, (2) no significant procedural changes may be introduced into the abortion procedure in the interest of research alone, and (3) no intrusion should be made that alters the duration of fetal life. All research involving the fetus should require the consent of the mother and the absence of any objection by the father, in view of his possible ongoing responsibility for the care of the fetus.

The Commission transmitted its report and recommendations on research involving the fetus on May 21, 1975. The recommendations were subsequently incorporated into DHEW [Department of Health, Education and Welfare] regulations without significant change. . . .[3]

What do moral theologians and moral philosophers have to say about fetal research and attempts to draw a line that determines when fetal destruction is permitted or prohibited? One deontologist, Princeton theologian Paul Ramsey, begins with the assumption that the "moment" of

3. "Summary of Activities," National Commission for the Protection of Human Subjects of Biomedical and Behavioral Research, May 17, 1978. Available from the Institute of Society, Ethics and the Life Sciences, Hastings-on-Hudson, N.Y. (also known as the Hastings Center).

biological conception is the beginning of human life. From that moment on, through all stages of fetal development, the unborn has the status and rights of a person. Ramsey maintains that fetuses are "protectable human beings."

By contrast, Harvard ethicist Sissela Bok denies that there is a natural biological point that confers human status and rights. According to her, a line must be drawn after which fetal life is protected, but this line is human-made. It is a line that we decide upon in light of all known biological facts and moral arguments. When asked "When does a developing fetus become a person?" Bok was reported by the *New York Times* to have responded as follows:

"I think that's a wrong question to ask," she said. "People have become simply mesmerized by that question, and it's really a question that has no answer. Because we are, after all, talking about something that is biologically 'human' not only after fertilization, but before—the ovum cell and sperm cells are certainly both living and human even before they meet.

"But if we are talking about 'personhood,' then I think it is impossible to speak of the fertilized egg, early in gestation, as 'a man,'" she continued, "although I realize that some theologians and others do. . . . It's as if one were to have to contemplate having funerals for two- or three-month fetuses that had miscarried or investigations for murder each time a fetus died *in utero* for reasons that weren't completely clear."

What it is essential to do, suggested Dr. Bok, is to draw a line—"an artificial line, admittedly, because as I said, nature hasn't provided us with a biological one"—at some point early in pregnancy and to say that beyond that stage of development no experimentation will be allowable. The line must, she stated, be drawn at a time in pregnancy when there can be no question whatsoever about the possible viability of the fetus to be used as a subject in biomedical research. "I think," she added, "that we'll always have to be very careful anyhow, and that it will be essential for us to continue having experimentation committees that can oversee and regulate all proposals for this kind of research."[4]

Present federal regulations regarding fetal research allow experimentation up to twenty weeks of gestation, or, presumably, before viability, that is, before the fetus could be kept alive outside of the woman's womb. (In passing, we must note that medical developments enable medical personnel to keep fetuses alive outside the womb at earlier and earlier stages.) The potential benefits of fetal research provide compelling reasons for many people who accept the inevitable fetal destruction. Certainly, it is *legally* acceptable, being within current guidelines of an agency of the federal government, the Department of Health and Human Services. But if fetal destruction in the course of experimentation can be justified up to

4. From Maggie Scarf, "The Fetus as Guinea Pig," *New York Times Magazine*, October 19, 1975.

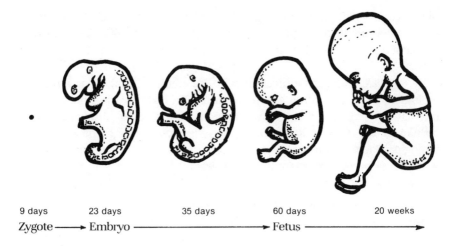

9 days   23 days   35 days   60 days   20 weeks

Zygote ⟶ Embryo ⟶ Fetus ⟶

twenty weeks after conception, then what about justifying fetal destruction up to twenty-four or even twenty-eight weeks of gestation for an abortion? (The Supreme Court decision of 1973 in *Roe* v. *Wade* makes abortion legal up to the end of the second trimester, or about twenty-eight weeks.)

ABORTION—THE EYE OF THE STORM

In the cases of *in vitro* fertilization (illustrated by the work of Steptoe and Edwards) and fetal research, some commentators justify the destruction of embryos and fetuses because they are nonviable and because the potential benefits to individuals and society through medical advances are great. But what about destruction of a fetus up to twenty-eight weeks of gestation, for *whatever private reasons* the woman who is carrying the fetus may have? According to current law, she need not give any reasons, her husband may not veto her decision; nor may her parents, regardless of her age. If fetal destruction up to twenty weeks is justified in the course of fetal experimentation, what could be wrong about a woman wanting an abortion up to twenty-eight weeks after conception?

Abortion is the issue that touches most of us personally, even within our own families. Abortion has been practiced throughout human history, whether legally permitted by a particular society or not. In the United States, the Supreme Court has legalized abortion in order to preserve a woman's right to a private decision about her pregnancy. In its famous decision in *Roe* v. *Wade,* the Court explicitly stated that it would not answer the central moral dilemma posed by abortion. The decision said that a woman, in consultation with her physician, may elect to have an abortion within certain limits. If she makes her decision within the first three months of her pregnancy, under the law the state may not interfere. During the second three months of pregnancy, the state may regulate aspects of the medical setting that can affect the mother's health by requiring, for example, that the procedure be performed in a qualified hospital or clinic. In the last three months of pregnancy, the state can intervene to protect the life of the fetus. In short, as pregnancy progresses, the state's interest increases to protect the life of the mother and the fetus, once it is within the range of viability. The Supreme Court said that "viability is usually placed at about 7 months (28 weeks), but may occur earlier, even at 24."

Subsequent court decisions have dealt with related matters. In the *Danforth* decision of 1976, it was ruled that a father could not overrule a decision made by the woman with her physician. The court again saw abortion as a woman's private decision in consultation with her doctor. In this matter, she has a right to noninterference.

Clearly the law and the sentiment of those who support access to abortion are on the side of the woman's privacy of decision. But two medical developments, specifically *genetic testing* and *prenatal diagnostic techniques,* force us to seek clarification of the degree of privacy and noninterference of a woman.

Genetic screening provides information to parents about the probabilities of their being carriers of certain inheritable diseases. Even if a man or woman is not affected, he or she can still be a *carrier.* Genetic testing techniques, which became available as early as 1969, enable parents to know whether they are carriers of recessive genes and to know also the probabilities of their having children who are carriers or, worse, are actually affected. Having this information that they are carriers, parents generally are more likely to ask for amniocentesis or some other prenatal diagnostic procedure. Amniocentesis can tell whether a particular fetus is affected and it can do so early enough to allow the option of legal abortion.

These same testing procedures can provide other kinds of information, such as the gender of the fetus. This raises a new problem: what about cases where a woman wants to abort a fetus because she has been told it will be a girl when she really wanted a boy, or vice versa? Does the doctor or society, through governmental guidelines and laws, have an obligation to qualify and limit the woman's currently accepted right to a private decision regarding abortion on grounds that a reason may be "trivial" or even "immoral"?

John C. Fletcher, assistant for bioethics to the director of the clinical center of National Institutes of Health, contends that, although he personally believes that gender selection is not a compelling reason for abortion, the legal rules defined by the Supreme Court clearly state that a woman's

Table 2   Chronology on Abortion Issue

Jan. 22, 1973: In Roe v. Wade, on a 7-to-2 vote, the Court legalizes abortion nationwide for the first time. Basing its ruling on a woman's right to privacy, the Court says a decision to have an abortion during the first three months of pregnancy must be left to the woman and her doctor. States may interfere in that decision only to protect the woman's health during the pregnancy's second trimester and may take steps to protect fetal life only in the third trimester.

Jan. 22, 1973: In Doe v. Bolton, on a 7-to-2 vote, the Court strikes down restrictions on facilities that can be used to perform abortions. Justice Blackmun writes for the majority.

July 1, 1976: In Planned Parenthood v. Danforth, the Court, 6 to 3, says states cannot give husbands of pregnant women veto power over the abortion decision. By a separate 5-to-4 vote, the Court says that neither can the parents of an unmarried young girl be given veto power.

Sept. 30, 1976: Congress imposes the Hyde Amendment, a spending restriction on Medicaid money made available for abortions. The appropriations measure is tacked onto the proposed budget for the Department of Labor and the then Department of Health, Education and Welfare. It takes effect Oct. 1.

Oct. 1, 1976: Cora McRae, a 24-year-old Brooklyn woman who suffers from varicose veins and blood clots, files a lawsuit. In September, she had sought an abortion at a Planned Parenthood facility and was told no Medicaid money was available because of the impending Hyde Amendment.

Oct. 22, 1976: Federal Judge John F. Dooling Jr. rules that the Hyde Amendment is unconstitutional and refuses to let the Federal Government enforce it. Mrs. McRae has her abortion, paid for by Medicaid, but meanwhile her lawsuit becomes a national "class action" with the rights of all women on welfare at stake.

June 20, 1977: In Maher v. Roe, on a 6-to-3 vote, the Court says that states have no legal obligation to pay for "nontherapeutic" abortions, but a definition of that term is not fully provided. The Court also stops short of saying whether such a financing obligation exists for "therapeutic" or "medically necessary" abortions.

June 29, 1977: The Supreme Court sets aside Judge Dooling's injunction, telling him to restudy his ruling in light of the Justices' June 20 decision.

Aug. 4, 1977: The Congressionally mandated spending restriction resumes, and Mrs. McRae's case returns to Judge Dooling's courtroom in Brooklyn. The judge hears from dozens of witnesses, sifts through thousands of pages of testimony and submissions, then deliberates for 13 months.

Jan. 9, 1979: In Colautti v. Franklin, reached by a 6-to-3 vote, the Court reaffirms its intention to give physicians broad discretion in determining the timing of "fetal viability"—when a fetus can survive outside the mother. States may seek to protect a fetus that has reached viability, but that determination is up to physicians, not courts or legislatures.

July 2, 1979: In Bellotti v. Baird, on an 8-to-1 vote, the Court elaborates on its parental consent decision of 1976, saying that states may be able to require a pregnant minor to obtain one or both parents' consent to an abortion if state law provides an alternative procedure, such as letting the minor seek consent of a judge instead.

Jan. 15, 1980: Judge Dooling issues a 622-page ruling once again striking down the Hyde Amendment.

Feb. 19, 1980: The Supreme Court refuses to postpone the effect of Judge

Table 2   (*Continued*)

Dooling's order to resume Federal financing for "medically necessary" Medicaid abortions, and such Government payments immediately are made available. On the same day, the Justices say they will add the McRae case to one from Chicago in which they had already agreed to rule on the Hyde Amendment's constitutionality.

June 30, 1980: In Harris v. McRae, on a 5-to-4 vote, the Court rules that the Federal Government and individual states have no legal obligation to pay for even medically necessary abortions.

Source: New York Times, July 1, 1980. © 1980 by The New York Times Company. Reprinted by permission.

decision about her pregnancy is private. A woman is not required to state her reasons when she requests an abortion.[5] James Childress, professor of Religious Studies at the University of Virginia, believes that Fletcher has overlooked something in the Supreme Court decision. The court emphasized that a woman's decision is to be made in consultation with her physician. The physician *is permitted to inquire* into the woman's reasons for an abortion. Childress also argues that physicians are not required to perform prenatal testing, even though they are probably required by law to inform the mother that such testing exists. Finally, Childress points out that the physician's own conscience is involved here, and that he or she is not morally bound to violate personal conscience by providing such diagnostic services, or, for that matter, by providing an abortion.[6]

Some who accept a woman's right to a private decision have difficulty accepting abortions of fetuses with genetic disorders. They have even greater difficulty accepting an abortion for the reason of wanting a child of the opposite sex. The private decision has *limits* to its privacy, they say. They argue that the fetus has a "right to life" that is at least equal to the woman's rights. Others argue that the woman's right to a private decision, for whatever reasons she chooses to discuss or keep to herself, is based on her being the one person primarily responsible for the birth and future of the child, as well as for her own well-being. What, if any, are the limits to privacy this society should accept regarding abortion decisions? At this point, you may want to review the situation illustrated in the case of Melinda Allen.

Suppose that you were told with certainty that your offspring would be seriously abnormal if born. Would you consider abortion? As a result of prenatal diagnosis, for example, suppose that you were told that the fetus

5. John C. Fletcher, "Prenatal Diagnosis for Sex Choice: Ethics and Amniocentesis for Fetal Sex Identification," *Hastings Center Report* 10 (February 1980): 15–17.

6. James F. Childress, "Prenatal Diagnosis for Sex Choice: Negative and Positive Rights," *Hastings Center Report* 10 (February 1980): 19.

was anencephalic, which means that the infant would have substantially no brain, and therefore almost certainly would die within the first few days after birth. Is abortion an alternative for you? On the other hand, maybe the fetus has been diagnosed as having Tay Sachs disease, a genetic disease most prominent in Eastern European Jews characterized by a normal early childhood, followed by progressive deterioration of the central nervous system, with death usually occurring by the teenage years. Somewhat less serious is a diagnosis of Down's syndrome. Children with Down's syndrome generally have an IQ of fifty to eighty, clearly abnormal. They can be trained in some cases to hold simple jobs and are famous for being happy, and they may live into adult life. Still, the children require very special care while growing up, and some supervision throughout their lives. Would you consider abortion of a fetus affected with Down's syndrome? Where do you draw the line on morally defensible abortions? Referring back to chapter one, how might you morally justify the line you have drawn?

The child, five inches long, with eyes, nose, mouth, hands and feet seemed very active. Martha sat feeling the imprisoned thing moving in her flesh, and was made more miserable by the knowledge that it had been moving for at least a week without her noticing it than by anything else. For what was the use of thinking, of planning, if emotions one did not recognize at all worked their own way against you? She was filled with a strong and seething rage against her mother, her husband, Dr. Stern, who had all joined the conspiracy against her.

—Doris Lessing,
A Proper Marriage

ECONOMIC BARRIERS TO ABORTION AND PRENATAL PROCEDURES

There are other ways to control access to abortion, specifically through the allocation of government money to fund abortions for poor women. This issue has spawned protracted political and moral debate in recent years. The availability of Medicaid or other government funds plays a leading role in providing access to abortion or, for that matter, any other prenatal medical procedure. These are politically controversial issues, and are likely to remain so in coming decades. How these issues are resolved is an important factor in the working consensus with which this society is struggling. They are discussed further in chapters 6–8.

THE REMAINING AGENDA

One could argue that abortion and other prenatal diagnostic procedures, as well as the laws and guidelines that prohibit or permit these kinds of procedures, remain controversial because we are morally uncertain about the value and rights of human beings. Lack of clarity about the moral status of the fetus before birth contributes to the social controversy. Some people assume that the Supreme Court decision of 1973 settled the abortion question and that other court decisions and guidelines of federal agencies in the 1970s settled the questions surrounding other prenatal medical procedures. However, ongoing social controversy and the unsettled reaction you (and others) may have had to situations such as that of Melinda Allen indicate that all aspects of these complex questions are far from settled.

Some continuing issues are:

1. How completely private *is* a woman's decision regarding abortion?
2. Ought society to provide funds to poor women to allow them equal access to abortion, prenatal diagnosis, and genetic screening?
3. Is there a sure consensus that "viability" is the line before which the woman's prerogative prevails and after which the fetus should be protected? Does it matter that science is moving the stage of viability closer to the time of conception?
4. As more information about a fetus becomes available to men and women while the fetus is still within the range of legal abortion, should limits be put on parents' decisional authority?

Beneath the social controversy lie questions that some say remain crucial because of the moral ambiguity of our society on this issue and because of continuing medical developments.

- What criteria of humanhood make a biological being a person—conception? some other point in fetal growth, such as "viability"? birth? consciousness?
- Where is the line in fetal development that demarcates the beginning of a fetus's status as an entity with human status and rights? Can such a line be drawn?
- What rights of the fetus and woman must be protected and, correspondingly, what are society's obligations to each?

In this chapter we have attempted to lead you along the full range of decisions to be made by individuals and this society in response to these questions. The selected readings that follow immediately will provide some background reading in primary sources; the annotated bibliography will provide established and recent reconsiderations of the crucial questions before us.

SELECTED READINGS
Life Begins at Conception[7]

If a spermatozoon is destroyed, one destroys a being which had a chance of far less than 1 in 200 million of developing into a reasoning being, possessed of the genetic code, a heart and other organs, and capable of pain. If a fetus is destroyed, one destroys a being already possessed of the genetic code, organs, and sensitivity to pain, and one which had an 80 percent chance of developing further into a baby outside the womb who, in time, would reason.

The positive argument for conception as the decisive moment of humanization is that at conception the new being receives the genetic code. It is this genetic information which determines his characteristics, which is the biological carrier of the possibility of human wisdom, which makes him a self-evolving being. A being with a human genetic code is man.

This review of current controversy over the humanity of the fetus emphasizes what a fundamental question the theologians resolved in asserting the inviolability of the fetus. To regard the fetus as possessed of equal rights with other humans was not, however, to decide every case where abortion might be employed. It did decide the case where the argument was that the fetus should be aborted for its own good. To say a being was human was to say it had a destiny to decide for itself which could not be taken from it by another man's decision. But human beings with equal rights often come in conflict with each other, and some decision must be made as to whose claims are to prevail. Cases of conflict involving the fetus are different only in two respects: the total inability of the fetus to speak for itself and the fact that the right of the fetus regularly at stake is the right to life itself.

"Life Never Begins—It Is Only Passed On"[8]

Another basic issue is raised between those who look at life phenomena episodically and those who view them epigenetically. This is a big-word way of saying that the question is: Is human life an event or a process? Or death, for that matter. Is the fetus, for example, a pattern or chain of incidents (fertilization, implantation, viability, and so on) or is it a pattern of development on a continuum? As Cyril Means has remarked a live human sperm and egg exist *before* fertilization; all that occurs is that two squads of twenty-three chromosomes each form up a platoon of forty-six, but "there is no more human life . . . than there was before." In human reproduction, the point is, life never begins—it is only

7. Excerpts from John T. Noonan, *The Morality of Abortion: Legal and Historical Perspectives* (Cambridge, Mass.: Harvard University Press, 1970), p. 57.

8. Excerpts from Joseph Fletcher, *The Ethics of Genetic Control* (Garden City, N.Y.: Doubleday, Anchor, 1974), pp. 142–43.

passed on by means of conception. Biology shows us that the process principle is the right one.

Even fertilization is a process—it takes at least two hours to complete the union of sperm and ovum. We simply cannot speak of the "moment" when life or death or mind or anything else biotic "occurs." They are not occurrences. All talk about a "human being" occurring at "the moment of conception" is old wives' talk. It is possible, presumably, to simply assert that the "soul" is "infused" at some point into a fetus in a single moment, but this is because there is no possible way to check it out. Nobody has ever seen one.

A person or personality is certainly not merely a quick event or episode. It takes many years to assemble a personality. A newborn baby starts excitingly soon to take on and store away the makings of a person, but even so it takes a long time. It is a process that starts at birth with whatever genetic constitution it has been physically formed by but it takes a considerable continuum to show results. Even the "switchboard" of the cerebral cortex needs several years of infancy and childhood to get the "wires" of the nervous system and brain "hooked up" for adequate human performance and growing up.

Whose Life Should Prevail?[9]

A *discussion of abortion* can help us understand what a right to life *is*. This is true even if we hold, as I do, that human beings have rights to life, but that fertilized ova do not have such rights.

A right to life includes more than merely being left alone; it also includes being able to acquire what one needs to live. Anyone who recognizes the right to life of a human child acknowledges this. One cannot simply leave a baby alone, unattended, to fend for himself or herself. One must see to it that babies have the necessary food, shelter, and so on. Access to what they need to live must also be included in the rights to life of adults, although this requirement is often overlooked, especially by so-called libertarians, who suppose that we respect persons' rights to life by merely not attacking them.

Abortion should be seen, not as an *attack* on the fetus, but as a refusal to provide it with what it needs to live. This refusal ought not to be made toward those who *have* rights to life. But who, then, has rights to life, and what do such rights require? Unfortunately, we do not now recognize the rights to life of vast numbers of human beings, both children and adults. They die of starvation, lack of medical care, and lack of basic necessities because those who could assure them what they need fail to recognize the rights to life of these people. And rights to life are not unlimited: Even where the basic minimum requirements of food, shelter, and medical care are provided through governmental arrangements that tax those lucky enough to have more than they need to provide for those who would otherwise die, rights to life do not give persons valid claims to unlimited amounts and kinds of resources. Thus no matter how much a person may need a new lung or kidney, he may have no right to one. And there are certainly limits to

9. Excerpts from Virginia Held, "Abortion and Rights to Life," in *Bioethics and Human Rights,* ed. Elsie Bandman and Bertram Bandman (Boston: Little, Brown, 1978), chapter 11.

what society should do in the way of mobilizing resources to deal with the right to life of someone with a rare disease, just as there are limits to what society should do to assure a citizen's right not to be attacked.

So rights to life sometimes are not recognized at all, and they are always recognized to have limits. Assuring rights to life often requires the efforts as well as the forbearance of others. But what about abortion?

It seems obvious that any discussion of abortion that fails to include a recognition that being pregnant and giving birth is an enormously exhausting and painful kind of labor does not even need to be given further attention. And yet we still hear discussion after discussion that fails to pay the slightest attention to the role of the woman, beyond referring to her "convenience." In all the vast literature on the subject of abortion, the most consistently overlooked consideration is: What does a woman do and feel when she makes a baby? Babies do *not* make themselves; women make babies. Yet this fact is ignored over and over, as the fertilized ovum is shown turning, as if by itself, into an embryo and then a fetus and then a baby and finally a grown human being.

The first thing we have to do in discussing abortion, then, is to bring clearly into the picture the woman who is making the embryo grow and, by expending a great deal of energy and pain, giving birth and producing a baby. Then the question is: What can justify requiring that she do so, against her will, either legally or morally? . . .

Many of those who strongly oppose abortion would not consent to the view that people should be forced to use their bodies for the sake of those in need of them, as in compulsory blood donation or skin grafts. They would not agree that persons should be compelled to do forced labor for others in need, such as for the poor. Except with respect to a woman's ownership of her own body, they have highly developed notions of the sanctity of private property. Although taxation is much less of a curb on liberty than is being forced to do a specific kind of labor, many opponents of abortion even oppose the level of taxation that would be necessary to allow those who are already human beings and fellow citizens to continue to live. The inconsistencies in such positions are startling. . . .

Our rights to own our own bodies are clearly not absolute. Our bodies are not possessions with which we can do whatever we like. Of course we do not have a right to use our bodies to attack and coerce other people as we please. And if a small child is hungry and needs to be fed, and you are her parent, the child has a legitimate claim to have you use your body to feed her. If a small child wants to climb on you, and you are his parent, I doubt that you would think, "get off my property." If the argument that a woman has a right to own her own body has been successful in persuading some judges and others that women should be legally allowed to decide whether to bear children or not, I cannot greatly regret that the argument has been used. But I do regret that the argument about the sanctity of private property is the one that touches so many, since it seems to me one of the weakest of the abortion debate. . . .

The view that the early products of conception can be considered persons with any sort of entitlement to life cannot be supported by any arguments that do not dissolve into myths when examined impartially. Religious myths have long influenced the debate by *conferring* personhood on such entities "from the moment of conception." Although believers should be free to consider the early products of conception "persons" on religious grounds if they wish, there are the strongest possible moral arguments against allowing such religious views to be imposed on those who do not believe them. More recently, for some people, genetic codes have taken the place of souls as the essential element of personhood. It has been argued that since the fertilized ovum contains the genetic code for a human being, the entity containing it has a right to life. But any number of cells contain genetic codes from which human beings could, with appropriate technology, be formed, as in cloning. The special status of the fertilized ovum thus disappears.

If we think personhood depends on aspects of human entities other than their possession of a genetic code, as any plausible view demands, we must admit that the early products of conception resemble sperm and ova more nearly in all relevant respects than they resemble babies. Then it seems arbitrary to claim that our moral concern, and our legal protection, should extend to zygotes but not to the billions and billions of spermatozoa wasted every day through masturbation. . . .

However, the nearer a fetus approaches the normal stage of birth, the more nearly it is entitled to consideration comparable in allowing the prohibition of abortion in the third trimester, except when necessary to preserve the life or health of the mother. It is also possible to imagine circumstances in which a society could justifiably require women to bear children: for instance, if birthrates fell to such a low level that the society was threatened with extinction. However, forbidding abortion would still be one of the worst ways to bring about an increased population. There are many ways to encourage women to have more children, such as making the burdens of child care and child support less severe for parents, particularly mothers. These arguments are especially relevant for certain groups who oppose abortion because they wish the numbers of members of their group to grow, or because they want enough babies of a certain kind to be available for adoption.

It is sometimes argued that if we allow abortion, we contribute to a disregard for life, and this disregard will spread to the weak and helpless of any age. It may be argued, on the contrary, that the all too common fixation on the fetus breeds excessive callousness toward the suffering of actual human beings. Making abortion illegal does not significantly reduce its occurrence; instead, it causes large numbers of women to die of complications from illegal abortions. In the Scandinavian countries where abortion has been permitted for some time, the care and concern for children and adults in need is among the best; in Nazi Germany, on the other hand, there were extremely strict laws against and harsh penalties for abortion.

We should, most certainly, have more concern for rights to life than we now have. But we should try to assure, as well, that such concern is directed toward those who need and deserve such concern and is not deflected into a campaign to impose forced labor on women for the sake of entities that have no such rights.

ANNOTATED BIBLIOGRAPHY
Books and Articles

Brody, Baruch. *Abortion and the Sanctity of Human Life: A Philosophical View.* Cambridge, Mass.: MIT Press, 1975. A thorough, book-length treatment of virtually all the moral problems of abortion mentioned in the literature. Brody writes from a conservative perspective.

English, Jane. "Abortion and the Concept of a Person." *Canadian Journal of Philosophy* 5 (October 1975): 233–43. The author casts serious doubt on whether the concept of personhood is sufficiently well-delineated to help resolve moral problems of abortion (as many writers have claimed it to do so).

Feinberg, Joel. "Abortion." In *Matters of Life and Death,* ed. Tom Regan. New York: Random House, 1980. A comprehensive and reasoned approach to almost all of the philosophical problems of abortion by a leading American philosopher who inclines toward liberal positions.

King, Patricia. "The Juridical Status of the Fetus: A Proposal for Legal Protection of the Unborn." *Michigan Law Review* 77 (August 1979): 1647–87. A lawyer takes a fresh look at the wide variety of moral and legal issues concerning the fetus. She argues for conclusions in many ways paralleling *Roe v. Wade*—but not for the reasons given by the U.S. Supreme Court.

Noonan, John T., Jr. *A Private Choice: Abortion in America in the Seventies.* New York: Free Press, 1979. The latest work by perhaps the best-known conservative writer on the subject of abortion. The author is a professor of law and argues that the law has been subverted for extralegal purposes in the instance of abortion.

Anthologies

Cohen, Marshall, Thomas Nagel, and Thomas Scanlon, eds. *The Rights and Wrongs of Abortion: A Philosophy and Public Affairs Reader.* Princeton, N.J.: Princeton University Press, 1974. A collection of difficult but significant articles by prominent moral philosophers.

Feinberg, Joel, ed. *The Problem of Abortion.* Belmont, Calif.: Wadsworth Publishing Company, 1973. The first and in some ways still the best collection on the subject. Philosophical and legal materials are featured.

Perkins, Robert, ed. *Abortion.* Cambridge, Mass.: Schenkman Publishing Company, 1974. An uneven anthology with some quite good pieces—especially the contribution by Sissela Bok.

Articles from the *Encyclopedia of Bioethics*

Abortion
  I. Medical Aspects *Andre E. Hellegers*
 II. Jewish Perspectives *David M. Feldman*
III. Roman Catholic Perspectives *John R. Connery*
IV. Protestant Perspectives *James B. Nelson*
 V. Contemporary Debate in Philosophical and Religious Ethics *Charles E. Curran*

VI. Legal Aspects *J. M. Finnis*
Person *A. G. M. van Melsen*

Literature

Walker, Alice. "The Abortion." In *You Can't Keep a Good Woman Down.* New York: Harcourt Brace Jovanovich, 1981. Imani, a black woman, records her changing self-image and relationships to her husband and daughter. Two abortions are important events. One was performed while she was still in school, before the 1973 Supreme Court decision, and the other was performed after the birth of her first child, when abortions are legal. The differences in the ways the two abortions are performed are of interest because of their social observations. But the larger context is the journey many contemporary women are making.

3

EUTHANASIA—DECISIONS ABOUT LIFE AND DEATH

AFTER HAVING WORKED AS A REGISTERED NURSE IN A HOSPITAL FOR EIGHT YEARS, RUTH Rowe left her job to care for her invalid mother, who demanded constant attention for fifteen years until her death. During that time, Miss Rowe had little social life, never married, broke with her religious faith, and became lonely and embittered. After her mother's death, Miss Rowe worked for an elderly physician and retired from practice when he did. Very soon thereafter, she discovered a lump in her left breast. Malignancy was confirmed and she had a mastectomy.

For the next three years Miss Rowe felt no further symptoms. Then she began to notice pain in her back and hip. She went back to the hospital where examination disclosed metastasis of the cancer to multiple bones. Her physician prescribed radiation therapy, which did relieve local pain, but in time pain and new lesions appeared in new locations. Her physician started chemotherapy, and, in addition, Miss Rowe received pills daily and intravenous injections frequently. Predicted side effects ensued, including nausea and vomiting and the loss of most of her hair.

It was at this point that Miss Rowe asked her physician to cease chemotherapy. "What's the use?" she asked. She also began to complain that the analgesics were not adequately controlling her pain. She asked her physician to supply her with several vials of morphine, which she could inject into herself to control pain. The physician was almost certain that Miss Rowe would accumulate the morphine until she had enough to hasten her death, but he complied with her request nevertheless. He also did not believe her cancer was in terminal stages, because breast cancer that spreads to bone can allow the patient to survive for years.

Miss Rowe refused help from social services, various support groups, and the ministry. Eventually, she saved up enough morphine for a lethal dose, took it all at once, and died at the age of 68.

Some Questions to Consider

1. Do you think Ruth Rowe had valid reasons for taking her own life? Did she have the *right* to do so? Do *you* have the right to do so?
2. What alternatives did she have?
3. Do you think the physician had any responsibility for her manner of death? Should he have confronted her directly about his suspicions concerning the morphine?
4. What obligations does a physician have to his or her patient in such cases? What obligations does a *patient* have to his or her *physician* in such cases? What mutual obligations were upheld or violated in this instance?
5. Should anyone have intervened in this case? Who? Why?
6. Should there be medical policies or laws that would permit an explicit arrangement between patient and physician in this kind of situation?

THE CHANGING DEFINITION OF EUTHANASIA

"Euthanasia" derives from a Greek word that means "good death." In classical times a good death was one that avoided prolonged suffering. In the first century B.C., Cicero might have spoken for many in the Greco-Roman world when he wrote, "What reason is there for us to suffer? A door is open to us—death, eternal refuge where one is sensible of nothing."

In our modern world the definition of euthanasia, and the issues around it, are becoming ever more complicated and challenging, for the principal reason that medical technology has given us the power to intervene and prolong life despite catastrophic illness or injury. The concept of euthanasia is now laden with matters of practical and ethical decision-making.

The questions are many, subtle, and undeniable. Are we bound by some ethical principle to forestall death, even at the expense of prolonged suffering? Under what circumstances, if any, should a patient be allowed to refuse lifesaving medical intervention? Is it proper for anyone else to make this decision for a patient? Family? Friends? Doctors? Should the financial or emotional limitations of the surviving family members be taken into account in some way? If a decision has been made to shorten suffering by accelerating death, is it "better" to withdraw treatment or to administer a lethal drug dosage?

We offer the following definition, which we believe includes the important nuances in current usage, of euthanasia:

Euthanasia—**putting to death or failing to prevent death in cases of terminal illness or injury; the motive is to relieve comatoseness,**

physical suffering, anxiety or a serious sense of burdensomeness to self and others. In euthanasia at least one other person causes or helps to cause the death of one who desires death or, in the case of an incompetent person, makes a substituted decision, either to cause death directly or to withdraw something that sustains life.[1]

MODERN MEDICINE CAN PROLONG LIFE . . . AND DYING

The motive for survival is so basic that many believe that hastening death can be understood only in the context of some mental illness. In fact, the effort to prevent and cure illness has provided one of the important driving forces for the development of medical science and technology. The progress of medicine and its associated technologies has been remarkable, a celebration of human ingenuity. Recently, an irony has emerged as medical chemistry and technology have given us unprecedented powers to prolong living. The problem, for those who deem it to be one, is that in the process of trying to prolong living we have developed the means to prolong *dying*, sometimes with the unintended consequences of extended pain, hopeless suffering, and loss of self-determination.

Until a few decades ago doctors stood helpless when a vital function of a patient's body began to fail. Now in many cases doctors can intervene to keep the patient alive. They can stop temporarily the progress of a disease, ameliorate damage to the body, or even replace a vital organ with a mechanical substitute. These technologies range from the simple to the sophisticated, from intravenous feeding and the use of antibiotics to resuscitation, dialysis, and the use of heart-lung machines.

Often used to help persons to recover from a disease or trauma, these technologies are seen as lifesaving measures. But when the new technologies were used to change dying into a prolonged process, some people began to doubt the blessing. Under these circumstances, dying may become a drawn-out series of degenerative changes. One vital function is repaired or replaced, and life continues at a reduced level of vitality and meaning. Later, another technology is applied and life continues at a still lower level of satisfaction. Finally, only by a very generous interpretation is a person still "alive." A terminal patient may be preserved in a comatose state for months or years by artificial means, with no hope of eventual recovery. Of course, people differ on the level of living they may find acceptable or burdensome. Some may endure great suffering to remain

---

1. Paraphrased from Tom L. Beauchamp and Arnold Davidson, "The Definition of Euthanasia," *Journal of Medicine and Philosophy* 4 (September 1979): 294–312.

alive while others may find unacceptable a lesser degree of suffering or even the thought of possible future suffering.

As long as a patient can be maintained in a condition that allows him or her to sustain an essential appreciation of life and the capability to make his or her own decisions, the issue of euthanasia usually does not emerge. Most patients and their families will endure pain and inconvenience, emotional strain and financial burdens for as long as they feel that life is "worth living" or that, in any case, there is a reasonable opportunity for recovery. Few question the desirability of using advanced means to resuscitate a patient in most situations. In a case of medical emergency, intravenous feeding may be the very means for patients to endure and recover to good health. Heart-lung and dialysis machines in most cases are welcomed means to sustain life.

Doubt arises when the patient seems to be losing ground despite these treatments and when the quality of life has become miserable; it is a matter of judgment and weariness and odds when a patient clearly foresees a long process of deterioration ahead, inevitably leading to death. The patient may come to prefer a swifter course. For family members and health care professionals, this can produce severe conflict for each person involved. Specifically, as with Ruth Rowe's physician, *a conflict arises between the instinctive and trained impulse to save life on the one hand, and on the other a wish to relieve or prevent unnecessary suffering.*

The success of medical science in maintaining life in even the most severely affected patient has contributed heavily to the current interest in euthanasia. For patients and families who have experienced similar situations firsthand, for others who have heard or read about these new kinds of problems, and for physicians and other health care professionals involved, there is fresh interest in the moral and legal aspects of euthanasia. Prolonged dying can include protracted pain and can lead to a patient's loss of competence to make decisions about his or her fate. This loss of competence in turn shifts decision-making about terminal care to the physician and family. Traditionally, these concerns about suffering, self-determination, and the duties of health care professionals when death seems imminent have been included under the topic of euthanasia.

WHEN THE PATIENT WANTS TO DIE

Once upon a time, pneumonia was called "the friend of the dying." Very often after it appeared in the course of a variety of terminal illnesses, death came rather quickly. The appearance of pneumonia in these circumstances still is common, but now we have the power to send away the friend of the dying.

What happens when a patient like Ruth Rowe wants to take her own life or refuse life-prolonging treatment? A number of our important cultural values come into play here. We respect the right of the individual's determination in many aspects of life, yet feel that it is normal and instinctive to wish to survive, and our culture dictates a profound respect for life.

If a patient wishes to die when his or her body is basically sound, then we go to extraordinary lengths to try to prevent the death. A suicidal but physically healthy individual is deemed to be mentally ill, neurotically or psychotically depressed. We intervene to try to eradicate the death wish. But what happens when the patient is not physically well and really does have a physical condition that he or she considers burdensome? Suppose further that the patient demonstrates a soundness of mind in other respects. How should we allow him or her to dictate his or her own death? This question is at the very heart of the current discussion of the controversy surrounding euthanasia.

It is more common these days than in the past to find cancer patients who wish not to undergo radical and prolonged treatment. Even dialysis patients (persons with kidney failure whose blood is rid of waste by a machine), many of whom can carry on some semblance of normal living routines, choose to reject or stop dialysis at a rate more than 100 times the suicide rate of the normal population. When a patient realizes that he or she cannot recover, and that he or she is imposing a tremendous financial and emotional burden on loved ones or on society, he or she may wish to die more quickly than standard treatment will allow.

EUTHANASIA DECISIONS ARE NOT LIMITED TO TERMINAL SITUATIONS

So far we have considered the case of Ruth Rowe, who at the end of a normal life span and faced with the prognosis of a terminal condition, wished to avoid prolonged suffering. Frequently the patient's wish, as we have pointed out, flies directly in the face of modern health care practices, which can do much to stall death. However, other kinds of situations requiring decisions regarding euthanasia can arise as well.

Some patients who wish to avoid prolonged suffering do not face terminal conditions. One example is the well-known case of a twenty-seven-year-old man who was burned over sixty-seven percent of his body in a freakish automobile accident in which the gas tank exploded.[2] Donald C.'s life was saved by a medical invention called the Hubbard tub. Before this invention, patients with such severe burns would have died from infection in the damaged skin. But daily dips in the Hubbard tub helped prevent infection in Donald C., and surgery corrected a few of the deformities to

2. Robert B. White and H. T. Engelhardt, Jr., "Case Studies in Bioethics, Case No. 228," *Hastings Center Report* 5 (June 1975): 9–10, 47.

Table 3

	Voluntary	Nonvoluntary
P A S S I V E	Mr. A has cancer. Dr. B recommends treatment that would prolong life. Mr. A refuses treatment.	Mr. A has cancer. Mr. A's family tells Dr. B not to use extraordinary means to prolong Mr. A's life. Dr. B follows the family's wishes.
A C T I V E	Mr. A has cancer. Mr. A asks Dr. B to administer a lethal drug. Dr. B does so.	Mr. A has cancer. Mr. A's family asks that he be given a lethal drug. Dr. B agrees and administers the drug.

his hands. In this particular situation, Donald wanted to cease treatment and go home, either to take his own life directly or to allow the inevitable infection to set in and kill him. His loss of sight and mobility and the pain of immersions in the Hubbard tub and bandaging were too much for him, he said. He explored legal means to obtain release from the hospital so he could go home to die. This case is mentioned to remind you that not all euthanasia decisions are faced by older persons in near-death situations. Some decisions, such as for infants with overwhelming disorders, are based on the "quality of life" the patients would know or on the impact of the patient's survival on the family and society. In the upcoming section about nonvoluntary euthanasia, these kinds of decisions for infants are discussed.

Table 3 may help to sort out the different kinds of euthanasia decisions that can be faced today. It uses the case of Mr. A, who has cancer, to represent all possible cases. From the generalizations this example permits, we will provide further distinctions in subsequent sections.

VOLUNTARY AND NONVOLUNTARY EUTHANASIA

The intensity of current concern about euthanasia has led specialists in medicine, philosophy, theology, and law to classify various types of euthanasia. We will discuss two of these distinctions, as they arise from the diagram above. The first distinction is between *voluntary* and *nonvoluntary* euthanasia, the second between *active* and *passive* euthanasia.

Voluntary decisions about death are those in which a competent and mature person requests or gives a formal consent to take a particular course of treatment or nontreatment. The decision expresses a person's conscious intent. Presumably, Ruth Rowe's decision reflected such deliberate intent. Some thinkers in the field conclude that such voluntary decisions ought to be honored in every case where euthanasia is desired. Others would honor such decisions only under some circumstances—for example, when patients have an agonizing terminal illness. In an influential article in favor of voluntary euthanasia, Glanville Williams[3] has argued that the patient should have complete liberty, including the right to have his or her life terminated. Williams can be said to represent those who believe that the right to avoid prolonged suffering is a primary right.

Yale Kamisar[4] has argued the opposite. He presents three primary arguments against voluntary euthanasia:

1. the diagnosis that a condition is terminal may be inaccurate, causing a person to make a decision for euthanasia on the basis of false or incomplete information;
2. the state of mind of seriously ill persons raises doubts about just how "voluntary" these decisions are;
3. any official support for voluntary euthanasia could constitute a "slippery slope" that could lead to abuses.

According to the slippery-slope argument, legalizing or permitting one action that is acceptable leads eventually to similar actions that are *un*acceptable. The only way to avoid the slippery slope is not to legalize or to permit the first, more acceptable practice.

Nonvoluntary decisions about death include situations in which a person is incompetent to make choices for himself or herself because of age, mental impairment, or even unconsciousness. The point is that the person who makes the decision about life and death is not the patient himself. Joseph Saikewicz, whose case study began chapter 1, exemplified a nonvoluntary decision made on the basis of his mental impairment. The famous Karen Ann Quinlan case was one in which her parents made the decision to remove life-support systems because she had been unconscious and hopelessly ill for many months. In nonvoluntary euthanasia the value questions concern who should be empowered to decide for an incompetent patient, and on what basis.

So far our discussion has considered questions about the fate of adults, especially those who are near death, but it is important to recognize that new medical technologies also have prompted questions about nonvolun-

---

3. See Glanville Williams, "'Mercy-Killing' Legislation—A Rejoinder," *Minnesota Law Review* 43 (November 1958): 1–12.

4. See Yale Kamisar, "Some Nonreligious Views Against Proposed 'Mercy-Killing' Legislation," *Minnesota Law Review* 42 (May 1958): 969–1042.

tary euthanasia for infants born with overwhelming medical problems. In the past these infants would have died early deaths. Now medical technology can intervene to save the infant's life, even though there may be no treatment for the serious birth defect. For example, consider babies born with spina bifida and hydrocephalus. These two separate conditions, which may occur in the same infant, are characterized by an opening in the back exposing the spinal cord and an accumulation of fluid in the head. Before 1957, it was common for such newborns to die fairly quickly. In that year, however, medical technology produced the Holter valve, which drains off the excess fluid that would otherwise cause death. Medicine now can save life, but still leaves the infant with paralysis, deformities of legs and spine, and no control over bowel or bladder. Furthermore, the maintenance and sterilization of the valve may require numerous operations. Using the Holter valve routinely with all infants born with hydrocephalus has saved lives, but in the process has produced much suffering and emotional and financial strain on their families.

Another well-known case of a nonvoluntary decision made for someone else—in this case a newborn—illustrates a substitute euthanasia decision made for an incompetent too young to make his own decision. Frequently referred to as the Johns Hopkins Hospital case,[5] it concerns a premature baby boy born to a couple in their mid-thirties. The infant had two significant medical problems: Down's syndrome (or mongolism) and duodenal atresia (an intestinal blockage). If surgery were performed to correct the intestinal blockage, the child would live but remain afflicted with Down's syndrome; if the surgery were *not* performed the child would die. The mother, supported by the father, refused to allow the operation. She said it would not be fair to the other children to raise a mongoloid child.

Cases of infant euthanasia poignantly demonstrate the importance of the concepts we accept or reject and of the laws and policies that we devise for society. They also demonstrate the importance of our second distinction, that between active and passive euthanasia. In the case of the child at Johns Hopkins Hospital, passive euthanasia was followed when the child was put off by itself and allowed to die. It would have been active euthanasia to administer a lethal drug to kill the child. Some argue that in such cases it is more humane to practice active euthanasia than to cause prolonged suffering and pain for the patient and emotional strain on attending health care personnel. Others argue that there are significant reasons not to allow active euthanasia, for example to prevent the potential result of killing other "undesirable" but viable infants and persons.

5. This case has been discussed in James M. Gustafson, "Mongolism, Parental Desires, and the Right to Life," *Perspectives in Biology and Medicine* 16 (Summer 1973): 529–57.

ACTIVE AND PASSIVE EUTHANASIA

While the distinction between *voluntary* and *nonvoluntary* decisions is fairly clear and straightforward, the distinction between *active* and *passive* is not. Is there any real difference between Donald C.'s going home and dying of subsequent, inevitable infection and his going home and using a weapon? Some would contend that perhaps it is even more humane to use the weapon.

The counterargument goes this way: A society may wish to permit passive euthanasia as a means to avoid the protracted pain and suffering that can accompany modern medical and health care practice; but to permit active euthanasia—especially nonvoluntary active euthanasia—could lead to abuses and possibly to permissive killing. For example, in the case of nonvoluntary active euthanasia decisions for infants, abuses could result in infants being killed for vague reasons. Later in this chapter we include an excerpt from the writings of James Rachels, who argues that if death is *intentionally caused* by doing something or withholding something there is no *morally* significant distinction to be drawn between an active means to death and a passive means to death. Both are alike on *intended means* to death; and both the intention and the result are the same—the death of the patient. Rachels argues the possibility that withholding treatment may cause the patient to suffer longer than if more direct action were taken. Specifically, he holds that "if one simply withholds treatment, it may take the patient longer to die, and he may suffer more than he would if more direct action were taken and a lethal injection given." Active euthanasia directly accomplishes the intent of the perpetrator(s) and may be more humane; passive euthanasia indirectly accomplishes the intent of the perpetrator(s) but may cause more suffering, he argues.

There are two primary kinds of responses to Rachels's argument. One could be labeled a deontological justification, which says that *there is an intrinsic modern difference* between active and passive euthanasia. The other could be called a utilitarian argument. Consider how these positions might be applied: one possible deontological response could be theological, the other nontheological. The theological response goes something like this: Life is a gift from a providential God. *Passive* euthanasia accepts the inevitability of death as God's will. *Active* euthanasia, on the other hand, sinfully takes the initiative of causing death by man's own decision and thus violates God's plan. A *non*theological deontological response reasons as follows: A distinction between active and passive euthanasia maintains medicine's duties to do good and to do no harm. The Hippocratic oath says, "I will use treatment to help the sick according to my ability and judgment, but I will never use it to injure or wrong them." This argument maintains that a physician must not deliberately be an agent of death.

Tom L. Beauchamp has written a utilitarian reply to James Rachels's claim that there is no difference between active and passive euthanasia. Beauchamp's work is also excerpted later in this chapter. At the basis of his argument is the proposition that a rule that allows only passive euthanasia may produce *fewer negative consequences* than a rule that permits active euthanasia. Producing fewer negative consequences would stand as justification of active euthanasia.

SOCIETY REACHES FOR POLICIES REGARDING EUTHANASIA

Euthanasia has taken on the proportions of an active social controversy. The sides in the controversy are not mutually exclusive or clearly drawn. Generally there is one group that expresses concern that medical technology might overwhelm human dignity, autonomy, and humane care for the dying. A different perspective is that medical and health care professionals and institutions should not be asked to become agents of death. For purposes of discussion here, we must assume that each position is valid.

The following letter is representative of recent concerns. It was received and printed in 1980 by the *New England Journal of Medicine*.

To the Editor: As one who has had a long, full, rich life of practice, service and fulfillment, whose days are limited by a rapidly growing, highly malignant sarcoma of the peritoneum, whose hours, days, and nights are racked by intractable pain, discomfort, and insomnia, whose mind is often beclouded and disoriented by soporific drugs, and whose body is assaulted by needles and tubes that can have little effect on the prognosis, I urge medical, legal, religious and social support for a program of voluntary euthanasia with dignity. Prolonging the life of such a patient is cruelty. It indicates a lack of sensitivity to the needs of a dying patient and is an admission of refusal to focus on the subject that the healthy cannot face. Attention from the first breath of life through the last breath is the doctor's work; the last breath is no less important than the first.

Consent by the patient with a clear understanding of this fact, by the patient's immediate family, by the family physician, lawyer, minister, or friend should violate no rules of social conduct. There is no reason for the erratic, painful course of the final events of life to be left to blind nature. Man chooses how to live; let him choose how to die. Let man choose when to depart, where, and what circumstances the harsh winds that blow over the terminus of life must be subdued.

Frederick Stenn, M.D.[6]
Highland Park, IL

6. Frederick Stenn, "A Plea for Voluntary Euthanasia," *New England Journal of Medicine* 303 (1980): 891.

To My Family, My Physician, My Lawyer and All Others Whom It May Concern

Death is as much a reality as birth, growth, maturity and old age—it is the one certainty of life. If the time comes when I can no longer take part in decisions for my own future, let this statement stand as an expression of my wishes and directions, while I am still of sound mind.

If at such a time the situation should arise in which there is no reasonable expectation of my recovery from extreme physical or mental disability, I direct that I be allowed to die and not be kept alive by medications, artificial means or "heroic measures". I do, however, ask that medication be mercifully administered to me to alleviate suffering even though this may shorten my remaining life.

This statement is made after careful consideration and is in accordance with my strong convictions and beliefs. I want the wishes and directions here expressed carried out to the extent permitted by law. Insofar as they are not legally enforceable, I hope that those to whom this Will is addressed will regard themselves as morally bound by these provisions.

Signed _____

Date _____

Witness _____

Witness _____

Copies of this request have been given to _____

_____

_____

It is obvious that medical sophistication has brought new options to doctors, patients, and the families of patients. All need practical, ethical, and moral guidance—some form of consensus about society's will in these matters. Accordingly, professional, religious, and social organizations regularly debate the issues and draft policy statements. Among such organizations have been the American Medical Association, the Catholic

Church, and various Protestant churches, as well as organizations such as Concern for Dying, which prepared and distributes the "Living Will."

The "Living Will" was developed in 1968 for people who wanted to leave written instructions "to my family, my physician, my lawyer, and all others whom it may concern" expressing their desire that extraordinary technologies not be used in the face of imminent death. In 1973 the American Medical Association issued a policy statement regarding euthanasia, and various religious groups throughout the 1970s did the same. Some state legislatures wrote "natural death acts" similar to California's, which was passed in 1976. These policy developments deserve consideration at this point.

The organization called Concern for Dying, which was founded as the Euthanasia Society of America, stated that their purpose was to assure patient autonomy in regard to treatment during terminal illness and to prevent the futile prolongation of the dying process and needless suffering by the dying. By contrast, consider the official position of the American Medical Association. The House of Delegates of the AMA adopted the position that "the intentional termination of the life of one human being by another—'mercy killing'—is contrary to that for which the medical profession stands and is contrary to the policy of the American Medical Association." The AMA statement goes on to say that the decision to cease "extraordinary treatment" is "the decision of the patient/family."

The AMA statement leaves the physician in the undefined role of "advisor." It does not necessarily contradict the statement of the Concern for Dying group. The two statements do, however, put different emphases on different sides of the dilemma. The Concern for Dying statement emphasizes patient autonomy and legal protection for health care practitioners who cooperate with patients' wishes. The AMA statement emphasizes that the physician ought not be involved in the intentional termination of life, which (unlike Rachels) they construe as *active* killing. The first statement grows out of concern for increasing patient self-determination, especially in regard to cessation of life-sustaining medical treatment. The latter grows out of an *equally* valid concern that medicine and its practitioners not become active agents of death. It could be said that the quest to balance these two concerns is the crux of the euthanasia dilemma. (This is an opportunity to reemphasize the fact that many of the dilemmas discussed in this book are not choices between "good and evil" or "right and wrong," but between at least two morally justifiable alternatives.)

In the 1970s some religious groups issued policy statements that expressed a position similar to that of the AMA. The Roman Catholic Church, for example, essentially supported the AMA position. Drawing on traditional moral theology and on a scholastic argument called "double effect," the Catholic Church reiterated a traditional position opposing active euthanasia. At the same time, the Catholic Church affirmed the importance of relief from suffering, even if the effect might be to shorten life.

The double-effect argument is a philosophical principle in Catholic moral theology. It states that whenever an action inescapably has two results, one bad and one good, it is morally permissible to intend an action for its *good* result and *allow* its *bad* result. There are qualifications (sometimes more than the three listed here):

1. the intention of the decision-maker must be to bring about the good result;
2. the action intended must be truly good, or at least not evil;
3. the good effect must produce at least as much good as the evil which accompanies it.

When applied to euthanasia, the double-effect rationale leads to a policy that condemns the active hastening of death but allows treatment for suffering even if the treatment produces an earlier death.

This excerpt from the Ethical and Religious Directives for Catholic Health Facilities conveys the Catholic position: "It is not euthanasia to give a dying person sedatives and analgesics for alleviation of pain, when such a measure is judged necessary, even though they may deprive the patient of the use of reason or shorten his life." A June 1980 "Declaration on Euthanasia"[7] issued by the Vatican condemns the direct taking of life. The declaration insists that all "normal" medical treatments should be used, but it allows the withholding of life-prolonging technology on the basis of considerations of suffering, burdensomeness, and excessive expense for family or community.

Positions like those of the AMA and the Catholic Church are derived from traditional allegiance to the Hippocratic oath and to a traditional interpretation of Jewish-Christian theology. Physicians in the school of Hippocrates (ca. 400 B.C.) pledged that they would "neither give a deadly drug to anybody if asked for it . . . or make a suggestion to this effect." From biblical times onward, Jewish-Christian theology has attempted to defer to God's will in matters of life and death. This position says that man is created in the image of God, the breath of life is breathed into humankind by God himself, and we are divinely commanded not to kill; therefore no human being has the right to kill another person, directly or indirectly.

Some other churches have articulated positions that could be viewed as more permissive than that of the Roman Catholic Church, and they em-

7. Sacred Congregation for the Doctrine of the Faith, "Declaration on Euthanasia," reported and excerpts published in the *New York Times,* June 27, 1980.

phasize patient self-determination to make decisions to refuse treatment. Typical of these positions is that of the United Methodist Church, which says, "We assert the right of every person to die in dignity, without effort to prolong terminal illness merely because the technology is available to do so." Another example is the position adopted by the United Church of Christ: "When illness takes away those abilities we associate with full personhood . . . we may well feel that the mere continuance of the body by machine or drugs is a violation of their person. . . . We do not believe simply the continuance of mere physical existence is either morally defensible or socially desirable or is God's will."[8]

Another kind of policy statement was a model policy for hospitals prepared in 1976 by the Law and Ethics Working Group of the Faculty Seminar on the Analysis of Health and Medical Practices of the Harvard School of Public Health.[9] The purpose of the statement was to offer hospitals guidelines for establishing policy for Orders Not to Resuscitate (ONTR). The Working Group acknowledged two important problems. First, practices regarding ONTR vary from hospital to hospital, and even from physician to physician, and "there has been little open discussion . . . of the process by which a decision not to resuscitate is formulated." Second, they recognized that, "having witnessed impressive medical developments over the past 25 years, the health care community is now confronted with complex questions arising from interplay of two such developments, technological advances and the increased emphasis on the patient's role in decisions concerning his own health çare." Recognizing these two realities, the Working Group went on to recommend a procedure that attempts to balance "the general policy of hospitals to act affirmatively to preserve the life of all patients" with "respect for the competent patient's informed acceptance or rejection of treatment including cardiopulmonary resuscitation." The importance of the statement to us is that it demonstrates an attempt to draft a hospital policy to balance two equally valid concerns in terminal-care situations: preservation of life and self-determination of the patient.

Individuals, groups and institutions, and the society at large have not reached a consensus about euthanasia because the moral problem beneath the public discussion is a profound dilemma in the sense discussed in chapter 1: we see a choice between two alternatives with apparently valid justifications.

8. These and other denominational policy statements have been published by Concern for Dying, 250 W. 57th Street, New York, N.Y.

9. Mitchell Rabkin, Gerald Gillerman, and Nancy Rice, "Orders Not To Resuscitate," *New England Journal of Medicine* 295 (1976): 364–66.

EUTHANASIA AND THE LAW

So far, case law and statutory law in the United States protect a diversity of policies and points of view regarding euthanasia. While the law remains ambiguous on some points, we do seem to have developed a pattern that allows some kinds of euthanasia. A review of past cases indicates that on occasion the courts have upheld *voluntary* decisions made by competent persons who refuse medical intervention, even when it could prolong life. In other cases, it has upheld *nonvoluntary* decisions (made by others) for incompetent persons who, due to age or mental or physical condition, are unable to make their own decisions to refuse treatment.

In cases where courts have upheld the voluntary decisions of a competent person to refuse treatment, there often is reference to the decision in *Schloendorff* v. *Society of New York Hospitals:*[10] "Every human being of adult years has a right to determine what shall be done with his own body; and the surgeon who performs an operation without his patient's consent, commits an assault for which he is liable for damages." You can easily imagine how this dictum, literally construed, would apply to Ruth Rowe: she must be permitted to hasten her death by a morphine overdose. More questionable, of course, is whether her right to self-determination morally required the physician to supply her with the morphine in the first place.

It should also be noted that today no American physician has been prosecuted successfully for terminating the treatment of a dying patient (competent or incompetent), in cases where there was no apparent hope of recovery. Currently, if the patient or guardian encounters a physician who refuses to honor a request for refusal of treatment, there are only two choices: one is to change physicians, the other is to go to court.

Legislation regarding euthanasia has been enacted in several states. There are three general kinds of legislation now in effect or under consideration:

1. provisions to permit instructions (for example, "Living Wills") for terminal care;
2. protection of the right to refuse treatment, even lifesaving treatment;
3. legalization of active hastening of death.

The first type is exemplified by the 1976 Natural Death Act in California. Under this law the individual, doctor, and hospital are protected when honoring such a written request. At the time of this writing, nine other states have passed similar legislation. Typically, these laws leave unclear

10. *Schloendorff* v. *Society of New York Hospital,* 105 N.E. 92 (N.Y., 1914).

the exact role of the family in cases where the patient is not competent to make the decision.

Proposed legislation of the second type attempts to put into statutory law that which has been assumed in case law. Specifically, these laws seek to protect a person's rights to privacy and self-determination in making decisions about his or her own body. Some critics argue that this kind of legislation may, in fact, *inhibit* progress toward a sensible law, because when legislation attempts to get specific, it usually increases the burden on the physician to determine whether a tratment will *cure* the patient or only *prolong* his or her life.

Proposals of the third type to "legalize" active hastening of death (by injecting a lethal substance, for example) have been heard in the British Parliament and in a few state legislatures. None has ever become law.

The Heart asks Pleasure — first —
And then — Excuse from Pain —
And then — those Little Anodynes
That deaden suffering —

And then — to go to sleep —
And then — if it should be
The Will of its Inquisitor
The privilege to die —

—Emily Dickinson,
"The Heart asks Pleasure — first —"

CONCLUSION

The hope for "the privilege to die" when death's time has come is ancient. But modern medical developments have given us choices to make where in the past we simply attempted to accommodate fate. Although practiced in some societies at various times and places, euthanasia historically has been condemned wholesale in nations with Judeo-Christian roots. Discussion about euthanasia has come about recently, we believe, because modern medical developments have created situations which have the unintended result of prolonging pain and suffering. The health care practitioner is put in a delicate position in such situations. His or her commitment is to life. That commitment is an unchallenged presupposition by the profession, the patient, and the society, especially in its laws. Yet there are those specific situations in which a person like Ruth Rowe or the parents of the infant at Johns Hopkins Hospital refuse the medical procedures that could prolong life because they want to prevent the maintenance of what *they* deem to be a life not worth living.

In the ongoing attempt of society to discover an equitable balance between these two legitimate, compelling concerns, it is no longer adequate to be for or against euthanasia, construed as a blanket term covering all forms of euthanasia. (Nor is it helpful to label one kind of euthanasia as "mercy killing" or some other pejorative label.) Distinctions between voluntary and nonvoluntary, and active and passive, euthanasia are important because they can help us sort out what *forms* of euthanasia each of us individually and our society as a whole may want to permit.

Various bills presented in state legislatures, statements made by churches and professional organizations, and the stories of individual cases that catch our attention in the media are all part of our collective search for an informed, equitable policy. Pieces of that policy are still under assembly.

SELECTED READINGS
Active v. Passive—There Is No *Real* Difference . . .[11]

The distinction between active and passive euthanasia is thought to be crucial for medical ethics. The idea is that it is permissible, at least in some cases, to withhold treatment and allow a patient to die, but it is never permissible to take any direct action designed to kill the patient. This doctrine seems to be accepted by most doctors, and it is endorsed in a statement adopted by the House of Delegates of the American Medical Association on December 4, 1973:

> The intentional termination of the life of one human being by another—mercy killing—is contrary to that for which the medical profession stands and is contrary to the policy of the American Medical Association.
>
> The cessation of the employment of extraordinary means to prolong the life of the body when there is irrefutable evidence that biological death is imminent is the decision of the patient and/or his immediate family. The advice and judgment of the physician should be freely available to the patient and/or his immediate family.

However, a strong case can be made against this doctrine. In what follows I will set out some of the relevant arguments, and urge doctors to reconsider their views on this matter.

To begin with a familiar type of situation, a patient who is dying of incurable cancer of the throat is in terrible pain, which can no longer be satisfactorily alleviated. He is certain to die within a few days, even if present treatment is continued, but he does not want to go on living for those days since the pain is

11. Excerpts from James Rachels, "Active and Passive Euthanasia," excerpted by permission of the *New England Journal of Medicine* 292 (1975): 78–80.

unbearable. So he asks the doctor for an end to it, and his family joins in the request.

Suppose the doctor agrees to withhold treatment, as the conventional doctrine says he may. The justification for his doing so is that the patient is in terrible agony, and since he is going to die anyway, it would be wrong to prolong his suffering needlessly. But now notice this. If one simply withholds treatment, it may take the patient longer to die, and so he may suffer more than he would if more direct action were taken and a lethal injection given. This fact provides strong reason for thinking that, once the initial decision not to prolong his agony has been made, active euthanasia is actually preferable to passive euthanasia, rather than the reverse. To say otherwise is to endorse the option that leads to more suffering rather than less, and is contrary to the humanitarian impulse that prompts the decision not to prolong his life in the first place.

Part of my point is that the process of being "allowed to die" can be relatively slow and painful, whereas being given a lethal injection is relatively quick and painless. Let me give a different sort of example. In the United States about one in 600 babies is born with Down's syndrome. Most of these babies are otherwise healthy—that is, with only the usual pediatric care, they will proceed to an otherwise normal infancy. Some, however, are born with congenital defects such as intestinal obstructions that require operations if they are to live. Sometimes, the parents and the doctor will decide not to operate, and let the infant die. Anthony Shaw describes what happens then:

> . . . When surgery is denied (the doctor) must try to keep the infant from suffering while natural forces sap the baby's life away. As a surgeon whose natural inclination is to use the scalpel to fight off death, standing by and watching a salvageable baby die is the most emotionally exhausting experience I know. It is easy at a conference, in a theoretical discussion, to decide that such infants should be allowed to die. It is altogether different to stand by in the nursery and watch as dehydration and infection wither a tiny being over hours and days. This is a terrible ordeal for me and the hospital staff— much more so than for the parents who never set foot in the nursery.[a]

I can understand why some people are opposed to all euthanasia, and insist that such infants must be allowed to live. I think I can also understand why other people favor destroying these babies quickly and painlessly. But why should anyone favor letting "dehydration and infection wither a tiny being over hours and days"? The doctrine that says that a baby may be allowed to dehydrate and wither, but may not be given an injection that would end its life without suffering, seems so patently cruel as to require no further refutation. The strong language is not intended to offend, but only to put the point in the clearest possible way.

My second argument is that the conventional doctrine leads to decisions concerning life and death made on irrelevant grounds.

Consider again the case of the infants with Down's syndrome who need opera-

a. A. Shaw, "Doctor, Do We Have a Choice?" *New York Times Magazine,* January 30, 1972, p. 54.

tions for congenital defects unrelated to the syndrome to live. Sometimes, there is no operation, and the baby dies, but when there is no such defect, the baby lives on. Now, an operation such as that to remove an intestinal obstruction is not prohibitively difficult. The reason why such operations are not performed in these cases is, clearly, that the child has Down's syndrome and the parents and doctor judge that because of that fact it is better for the child to die.

But notice that this situation is absurd, no matter what view one takes of the lives and potentials of such babies. If the life of such an infant is worth preserving, what does it matter if it needs a simple operation? Or, if one thinks it better that such a baby should not live on, what difference does it make that it happens to have an unobstructed intestinal tract? In either case, the matter of life and death is being decided on irrelevant grounds. It is the Down's syndrome, and not the intestines, that is the issue. The matter should be decided, if at all, on that basis, and not be allowed to depend on the essentially irrelevant questions of whether the intestinal tract is blocked.

What makes this situation possible, of course, is the idea that when there is an intestinal blockage, one can "let the baby die," but when there is no such defect there is nothing that can be done, for one must not "kill" it. The fact that this idea leads to such results as deciding life or death on irrelevant grounds is another good reason why the doctrine should be rejected.

One reason why so many people think that there is an important moral difference between active and passive euthanasia is that they think killing someone is morally worse than letting someone die. But is it? Is killing, in itself, worse than letting die?

. . . But the Distinction Can Be Useful[12]

. . . I wish now to provide what I believe is the most significant argument that can be adduced in defense of the active/passive distinction. I shall develop this argument by combining (1) so-called wedge or slippery slope arguments with (2) recent arguments in defense of rule utilitarianism. I shall explain each in turn and show how in combination they may be used to defend the active/passive distinction.

(1) *Wedge arguments* proceed as follows: if killing were allowed, even under the guise of a merciful extinction of life, a dangerous wedge would be introduced which places all "undesirable" or "unworthy" human life in a precarious condition. Proponents of wedge arguments believe the initial wedge places us on a slippery slope for at least one of two reasons: (i) It is said that our justifying principles leave us with no principled way to avoid the slide into saying that all sorts of killings would be justified under similar conditions. Here it is thought that once killing is allowed, a firm line between justified and unjustified killings cannot be securely drawn. It is thought best not to redraw the line in the first place, for redrawing it will inevitably lead to a downhill slide. It is then often

---

12. Excerpts from Tom L. Beauchamp, "A Reply to Rachels on Active and Passive Euthanasia," in *Ethical Issues in Death and Dying*, ed. Tom L. Beauchamp and Seymour Perlin (Englewood Cliffs, N.J.: Prentice-Hall, 1978), pp. 246 ff. © 1975, 1977 by Tom. L. Beauchamp.

pointed out that as a matter of historical record this is precisely what has occurred in the darker regions of human history, including the Nazi era, where euthanasia began with the best intentions for horribly ill, non-Jewish Germans and gradually spread to anyone deemed an enemy of the people. (ii) Second, it is said that our basic principles against killing will be gradually eroded once some form of killing is legitimated. For example, it is said that permitting voluntary euthanasia will lead to permitting involuntary euthanasia, which will in turn lead to permitting euthanasia for those who are a nuisance to society (idiots, recidivist criminals, defective newborns, and the insane, e.g.). Gradually other principles which instill respect for human life will be eroded or abandoned in the process.

I am not inclined to accept the first reason (i). If our justifying principles are themselves justified, then any action they warrant would be justified. Accordingly, I shall only be concerned with the second approach (ii).

(2) *Rule utilitarianism* is the position that a society ought to adopt a rule if its acceptance would have better consequences for the common good (greater social utility) than any comparable rule could have in that society. Any action is right if it conforms to a valid rule and wrong if it violates the rule. Sometimes it is said that alternative rules should be measured against one another, while it also has been suggested that whole moral *codes* (complete sets of rules) rather than individual rules should be compared. While I prefer the latter formulation (Brandt's), this internal dispute need not detain us here. The important point is that a particular rule or a particular code of rules is morally justified if and only if there is no other competing rule or moral code whose acceptance would have a higher utility value for society, and where a rule's acceptability is contingent upon the consequences which would result if the rule were made current.

Wedge arguments, when conjoined with rule utilitarian arguments, may be applied to euthanasia issues in the following way. We presently subscribe to a no-active-euthanasia rule (which the AMA suggests we retain). Imagine now that in our society we make current a restricted-active-euthanasia rule (as Rachels seems to urge). Which of these two moral rules would, if enacted, have the consequences of maximizing social utility? Clearly a restricted-active-euthanasia rule would have *some* utility value, as Rachels notes, since some intense and uncontrollable suffering would be eliminated. However, it may not have the highest utility value in the structure of our present code or in any imaginable code which could be made current, and therefore may not be a component in the ideal code for our society. If wedge arguments raise any serious questions at all, as I think they do, they rest in this area of whether a code would be weakened or strengthened by the addition of active euthanasia principles. For the disutility of introducing legitimate killing into one's moral code (in the form of active euthanasia rules) may, in the long run, outweigh the utility of doing so, as a result of the eroding effect such a relaxation would have on rules in the code which demand respect for human life. If, for example, rules permitting active killing were introduced, it is not implausible to suppose that destroying defective newborns (a form of involuntary euthanasia) would become an accepted and common practice, that as population increases occur the aged will be even more neglectable and neglected than they now are, that capital punishment for a wide variety of crimes would be increasingly tempting, that some doctors would have appreciably reduced fears of actively injecting fatal doses whenever it seemed to them propitious to do so, and that laws of war against killing would erode in efficacy even beyond their already abysmal level.

A hundred such possible consequences might easily be imagined. But these few are sufficient to make the larger point that such rules permitting killing could lead to a general reduction of respect for human life. Rules against killing in a moral code are not *isolated* moral principles; they are pieces of a web of rules against killing which forms the code. The more threads one removes, the weaker the fabric becomes. And if, as I believe, moral principles against active killing have the deep and continuously civilizing effect of promoting respect for life, and if principles which allow passively letting die (as envisioned in the AMA statement) do not themselves cut against this effect, then this seems an important reason for the maintenance of the active/passive distinction. (By the logic of the above argument passively letting die also would have to be prohibited if a rule permitting it had the serious adverse consequence of eroding acceptance of rules protective of respect for life. While this prospect seems to me improbable, I can hardly claim to have refuted those conservatives who would claim that even rules which sanction letting die place us on a precarious slippery slope.)

A troublesome problem, however, confronts my use of utilitarian and wedge arguments. Most all of us would agree that both killing and letting die are justified under some conditions. Killings in self-defense and in "just" wars are widely accepted as justified because the conditions excuse the killing. If society can withstand these exceptions to moral rules prohibiting killing, then why is it not plausible to suppose society can accept another excusing exception in the form of justified active euthanasia? This is an important and worthy objection, but not a decisive one. The defenseless and the dying are significantly different classes of persons from aggressors who attack individuals and/or nations. In the case of aggressors, one does not confront the question whether their lives are no longer *worth living*. Rather, we reach the judgment that the aggressors' morally blameworthy actions justify counteractions. But in the case of the dying and the otherwise ill, there is no morally blameworthy action to justify our own. Here we are required to accept the judgment that their lives are no longer *worth living* in order to believe that the termination of their lives is justified. It is the latter sort of judgment which is feared by those who take the wedge argument seriously. We do not now permit and never have permitted the taking of morally blameless lives. I think this is the key to understanding why recent cases of intentionally allowing the death of defective newborns (as in the now famous case at the Johns Hopkins Hospital) have generated such protracted controversy. Even if such newborns could not have led meaningful lives (a matter of some controversy), it is the wedged foot in the door which creates the most intense worries. For if we once take a decision to allow a restricted infanticide justification or any justification at all on grounds that a life is not meaningful or not worth living, we have qualified our moral rules against killing. That this qualification is a matter of the utmost seriousness needs no argument. I mention it here only to show why the wedge argument may have moral force even though we *already* allow some very different conditions to justify intentional killing.

There is one final utilitarian reason favoring the preservation of the active/ passive distinction. Suppose we distinguish the following two types of cases of wrongly diagnosed patients:

1. Patients wrongly diagnosed as hopeless, and who will survive even if a treatment *is* ceased (in order to allow a natural death).
2. Patients wrongly diagnosed as hopeless, and who will survive only if the treatment is *not ceased* (in order to allow a natural death).

If a social rule permitting only passive euthanasia were in effect, then doctors and families who "allowed death" would lose only patients in class 2, not those in class 1; whereas if active euthanasia were permitted, at least some patients in class 1 would be needlessly lost. Thus, the consequence of a no-active-euthanasia rule would be to save some lives which could not be saved if both forms of euthanasia were allowed. This reason is not a decisive reason for favoring a policy of passive euthanasia, since these classes (1 and 2) are likely to be very small and since there might be counterbalancing reasons (extreme pain, autonomous expression of the patient, etc.) in favor of active euthanasia. But certainly it is a reason favoring only passive euthanasia and one which is morally relevant and ought to be considered along with other moral reasons.

ANNOTATED BIBLIOGRAPHY
Books and Articles

Childress, James F. "To Live or Let Die." In *Priorities in Biomedical Ethics*, by James F. Childress. Philadelphia: Westminster Press, 1981. Pp. 34–50. A clear and well-versed writer on ethical issues explores our responsibilities to treat or to let die in various circumstances. Balanced and judicious without opting for any polar position.

Devine, Philip E. *The Ethics of Homicide.* Ithaca, N.Y.: Cornell University Press, 1978. A strongly argued conservative account of the immorality of euthanasia practices. Detailed and probing argument—often technical.

McCormick, Richard A. "To Save or Let Die: The Dilemma of Modern Medicine." *Journal of the American Medical Association* 229 (1974): 172–76. An influential article by a liberal Roman Catholic writer. The article surprised many Roman Catholics at the time.

Rachels, James. "Euthanasia." In *Matters of Life and Death*, ed. Tom Regan. New York: Random House, 1980. A near-monograph development of many issues about euthanasia. Rachels develops the views found in this chapter in a broader setting.

Veatch, Robert M. *Death, Dying and the Biological Revolution.* New Haven: Yale University Press, 1976. One of the most distinguished books in the field by a clear writer. Veatch is equally concerned with issues of private choice and public policy.

Anthologies

Beauchamp, Tom L., and Perlin, Seymour, eds. *Ethical Issues in Death and Dying.* Englewood Cliffs, N.J.: Prentice-Hall, 1978. Chaps. 3 and 4. Some of the best materials on the rights of the dying and on euthanasia are found here in edited form.

Behnke, John A., and Bok, Sissela, eds. *The Dilemma of Euthanasia.* Garden City, N.Y.: Doubleday, Anchor, 1975. An uneven but nonetheless useful series of essays on a variety of topics. Accessible, inexpensive, and widely used.

Ladd, John, ed. *Ethical Issues Relating to Life and Death.* New York: Oxford University Press, 1979. A collection of difficult but probing essays that push forward the debate about euthanasia.

Articles from the *Encyclopedia of Bioethics*

Acting and Refraining *Harold Moore*
Aging and the Aged: Ethical Implications in Aging *Drew Christiansen*
Death and Dying: Euthanasia and Sustaining Life
  I. Historical Perspectives *Gerald J. Gruman*
  II. Ethical Views *Sissela Bok*
  III. Professional and Public Policies *Robert M. Veatch*
Double Effect *William E. May*
Infanticide *Michael Tooley*
Life: Value of Life *Peter Singer*
Life: Quality of Life *Warren Reich*
Life Support Devices: Philosophical Perspectives *A. G. M. van Melsen*
Pain and Suffering: Philosophical Perspective *Jerome Shaffer*

Literature

Beauvoir, Simone de. *A Very Easy Death.* New York: Warner Paperback Library, 1964. In her autobiographical record, Beauvoir follows the death of her aged mother. She reflects on her mother's dying in a modern hospital, her decision for surgery over a faster, less painful death for her mother and finally a nurse's comment that her mother died "naturally."

Audio/Visual

"Please Let Me Die." 30-minute film or videotape. Sale or rental available to limited audiences, Library of Clinical Psychiatric Syndromes, Department of Psychiatry, University of Texas Medical Branch, Galveston, Tex., 77550. Interviews with Donald C., whose case was discussed in this chapter.

"Who Should Survive?" 26-minute film. Sale or rental, Lowengard and Brotherhood, 12 Charter Oaks Place, Hartford, Conn., 06106. The Johns Hopkins Hospital case discussed in this chapter is considered from several perspectives.

4

DEATH AND PERSONHOOD

AT 42, BILL SAMUELS CONCENTRATED MOST OF HIS ENERGIES ON HIS JOB AS A TRAVELING salesman. His home base was Minneapolis, but with no family at home, and no other relatives in Minneapolis, work-related travel became a way of life. Several years ago he flew to Los Angeles and rented a car in order to make several important calls in southern California. The freeway accident involved four cars and a truck. Bill was taken unconscious to the emergency room of the nearest hospital. The examining physician discovered massive head injuries and multiple fractures. Bill required many transfusions and a respirator to maintain oxygenation. The doctor was encouraged by the fact that Bill's heart and kidneys were functioning normally.

In Bill's business suit, which had been cut away from him during the hurried initial examination, a nurse found a wallet that provided identification. She also found something unusual—a Uniform Anatomical Gift Card, which is a voluntary statement expressing the individual's own wish that his or her remains be used upon death for transplantation or research. Quickly, the hospital alerted the transplant team while attempts were being made to locate Bill's family. Bill himself was placed in the intensive care unit, and the chief of the transplant team was designated as his attending physician.

An electroencephalogram (brain-wave test) showed no brain activity. This confirmed what doctors had suspected—a massive insult to Bill's brain. The transplant team moved immediately to examine blood samples in order to determine Bill's tissue type. A survey of potential transplant recipients yielded two patients with end-stage kidney disease and one patient with terminal heart failure, all matching Bill's tissue type. These patients were notified to come to the hospital and stand by.

Finding no family contact in Minneapolis, the hospital called Bill's employer in an attempt to reach some relative. The employer knew only of an invalid mother in a nursing home. Doctors spoke with the mother's physician, who declared her incompetent to participate in any decision-making. The search for relatives seemingly was futile. After thirty-six hours the California doctors observed no clinical changes in Bill's condition; his encephalogram was still flat. He showed no spontaneous motion, no reaction to painful stimuli, and he still required the respirator. Meanwhile, the potential transplant recipients and their families maintained a vigil nearby. They questioned the doctors and nurses constantly about the circumstances. It was time for decisions to be made.

The attending physician consulted two other doctors, who concurred that "brain death" had occurred. The attending physician made his decision. He set into motion a complex ethical and technological drama that would have been almost unthinkable twenty-five years ago. Bill Samuels and all three recipients were moved into operating rooms. Bill's heart, still beating, and both kidneys were removed and transplanted into the waiting patients.

The next day Bill's sister, who had been notified of the accident by one of Mr. Samuels's co-workers in Minneapolis, arrived from Toronto. She was overwhelmed with sorrow and disbelief; then she was angry. Later she initiated legal proceedings. Her attorney argued several points:

1. Minnesota, Bill's home state, did not recognize "brain death" as a *legal* definition of death.
2. Further, under Minnesota laws, the remains of the deceased become the property of the next of kin—in this case, the property of his sister.
3. Finally, the lawyer argued that the hospital should not have appointed a member of the transplant team to be Bill's attending physician. He contended that this doctor's first allegiance was to patients needing organ transplants, and that the doctor could not have acted on behalf of Bill Samuels with a clear purpose.

The hospital and physicians countered that death occurred in the state of California, not Minnesota, and that local laws—which did recognize brain death—applied in this case. Further, they contended that the donor card gave a clear indication of the patient's wishes and that Bill's death had been determined by objective criteria and confirmed by two other physicians.

Some Questions to Consider
1. At the time Bill Samuels's organs were removed, was he dead or alive?
2. In your state, or similar legal jurisdiction, would Samuels have been considered dead or alive? What about in neighboring states?
3. In situations similar to this case, do you believe that a single doctor's informed medical judgment is sufficient to make such determinations of death or decisions about transplantation? Why yes? Why no?
4. How do you feel about organ transplantation? Do you believe a person's body is special in some way or ought its organs be used at the time of death for transplantations to waiting recipients or for some other beneficial cause?
5. What is lost at death that causes us to regard the person we have known as "gone"? Is it spontaneous breathing and heartbeat, artificially maintained breathing and heartbeat, consciousness, characteristics such as speech, reason, and similar traits that marked him or her as a living person? Or is it an entity such as the spirit or soul? Which *one* of these would you name and why?

WHEN IS A PERSON DEAD?

The mysteries of life and death, the dimly outlined entry and exit points for an individual's animated journey on earth, constitute some of our major preoccupations as a species. The beginning and ending of life take positions alongside love and striving to overcome obstacles as the major themes in our poetry and fiction, our graphic and musical arts, our worship and our ceremonies of celebration and mourning. Increasingly now, as a result of the new controls over life provided by medical advances, these issues are becoming salient ones in our official policies and laws.

In the second chapter we dealt with issues surrounding the *beginning* of life, issues such as abortion and conception *in vitro*. Underlying those issues is a concern to know the earliest stages at which we can regard a new life as fully "human," a new individual who properly should be considered a person from moral and legal points of view. Now we leap across the human life span to consider similar issues that attend the process or moment of dying. Considering that doctors know how to intervene in order to prolong some of the traditional "signs of life," it becomes a practical necessity to develop criteria for answering the question, "When is a person dead?"

Most of us first learned about dying from novels and the movies or television. Enemy soldiers, villains, cowboys, and gangsters tended to die in a rather simple and straightforward way. They toppled like trees, and if any attempt were made to confirm death, it consisted simply of listening for a heartbeat or touching the wrist to feel for a pulse. Sick or very old people often remained lucid to the end, whispering last words before expiring. Even before the doctor shook his head, everyone in the room knew that the patient had died. Today none of these traditional criteria would necessarily be accepted as an indication of death, and we have grown accustomed to reading more and more stories in the newspapers like the case of Bill Samuels.

The situation is thus very different today than it was in former times. In a modern medical facility, the normal progression of events in a "dying" patient often is subject to the kind of control that we have in stop-action photography. We have all seen the fascinating effects that can be achieved when a director stops a film at the moment when a bud begins to open into a flower or freezes a videotape replay at the moment a football touches the outstretched fingers of the receiver. To be sure, doctors do not have quite this much control over the processes they deal with, but still they can arrest the process of dying at certain key points. Intervening to slow down the process of dying provides time in which family and medical staff are required to make decisions. How long should the patient be held in his or her current condition? Are there alternative manipulations that should be considered? Is the patient suffering? After a loss of measurable brain activity, is the patient still a human being? Was Bill Samuels a human being before the transplant? After the transplant?

While maintaining a patient in the indefinite space between personhood and death, it is natural that we would begin to wonder exactly when, for practical, moral, or legal purposes, the patient really should be considered "dead."

DOES "BRAIN DEATH" ANSWER THE QUESTION?

We search for an answer because ethically we feel that we have to know. Attitudes, intense feelings, and practical responsibilities are involved in this decision. For so long as we believe that we still have grandmother, that "she" is there in the hospital bed, desperately ill, we operate according to one set of ethical principles. The moment that we believe that grandmother is *not* there, that her life is physically, biologically absent, we are prepared by our instincts and traditions to adopt entirely different attitudes and courses of action. Great moral and ethical importance attaches to a declaration of death.

In trying to establish criteria by which to determine death, much of the medical community has given special importance to "brain death"—an absence of brain wave activity associated with the living. We know that the cells of the brain, once dead, cannot be regenerated or replaced. Physicians reason that once the brain has lost the ability to animate and regulate the life systems of the body, then the situation is quite hopeless; except by artificial and external means, no semblance of "life" can be maintained in that body.

In 1968, an interdisciplinary group at Harvard University (an Ad Hoc Committee to examine the Definition of Brain Death) published a report which presented brain death as a proper "definition" of death.[1] The committee, whose purpose was to standardize what many physicians were already doing, presented four criteria which, if observed for twenty-four hours, would justify a pronouncement of death. These criteria are noted below:

1. *Unreceptivity and unresponsivity to external stimuli.* Stated simply, this means that the individual does not show any signs of awareness of sound, touch, etc.
2. *No spontaneous movements or breathing observed.* In other words, the only motion observed in the body is that which is produced by external manipulation; even breathing must be done by a machine.
3. *No reflexes.* Even severely ill or injured persons will demonstrate reflexes in the concentration of the pupils, for example, if there is sufficient life in the brain. This may be true even when the patient is entirely unconscious.

1. "A Definition of Irreversible Coma," a report of the Ad Hoc Committee of the Harvard Medical School to Examine the Definition of Brain Death, in *Journal of the American Medical Association* 205 (1968): 337–40.

4. *A flat encephalogram.* An encephalogram measures, through sensors attached to the skull, the minute electrical activity associated with the living brain. A flat encephalogram refers to the straight line produced on the instrument's recording paper when there is no wave activity at all.

The Harvard definition—often with slight modifications—has found its way into everyday policy and practice. Although this definition of death is by no means universal, it now is the basis of law in many states. Furthermore, its attraction has been enhanced because, unlike breathing and heart function, which sometimes can be reactivated after short stoppage or aided or replaced mechanically, cessation of brain activity is irreversible. It has been necessary for the medical and legal communities to formalize their views about death, if only because it is so expensive and so completely hopeless to sustain "life" after the loss of brain function. Doctors know from experience that they often can sustain a person in this condition indefinitely—just as Bill Samuels could have been, but was not. Some persons have been maintained with artificial heart and lung support without registering brain activity for months, some for years. These kinds of cases have contributed to the pressure to arrive at a moral and legal consensus regarding a uniform determination of death.

In the public deliberation that ensued after the Harvard "brain death" definition was published, an important distinction was made between the cessation of two different parts of the brain. Some believed that cessation of the neocortex part of the brain, the part that controls functions of speech, reasoning, and other "higher" human capacities, was sufficient to declare death. But others held that cessation of the "whole" brain was necessary; that is, the stem of the brain in which the centers for nonvoluntary functions such as breathing and body temperature regulation are controlled. The former group declared that once the "higher" functions ceased, the qualities that make a human being "human" had ceased irreversibly and, with them, the qualities that make each person unique. The latter group held, however, that medical technologies, as sophisticated as they are, could not predict irreversibility and that if spontaneous breathing and heartbeat continued, the patient ought not be declared dead. For example, under the first distinction, Karen Ann Quinlan would be considered dead, and under the second, alive. (You will need to keep this distinction in mind or return to it when we discuss the proposed "Uniform Determination of Death.")

LAW—THE LIFE AND DEATH OF RIGHTS

By its origins and its methods, medicine is a *science.* By definition, then, its purpose is to document and extend the definition of what is *possible,*

Table 4 Levels of the Definition of Death

Formal Definition: Death means a complete change in the status of a living entity characterized by the irreversible loss of those characteristics that are essentially significant to it.

Concept of death: philosophical or theological judgment of the essentially significant change at death.	*Locus of death:* place to look to determine if a person has died.	*Criteria of death:* measurements physicians or other officials use to determine whether a person is dead—to be determined by scientific empirical study.
1. The irreversible stopping of the flow of "vital" body fluids, i.e., the blood and breath	Heart and lungs	1. Visual observation of respiration, perhaps with the use of a mirror 2. Feeling of the pulse, possibly supported by electrocardiogram
2. The irreversible loss of the soul from the body	The pineal body? (according to Descartes) The respiratory track?	Observation of breath?
3. The irreversible loss of the capacity for bodily integration and social interaction	The brain	1. Unreceptivity and unresponsivity 2. No movements or breathing 3. No reflexes (except spinal reflexes) 4. Flat electroencephalogram (to be used as confirmatory evidence) —All tests to be repeated 24 hours later (excluded conditions: hypothermia and central nervous system drug depression)
4. Irreversible loss of consciousness or the capacity for social interaction	Probably the neocortex	Electroencephalogram

Note: The possible concepts, loci, and criteria of death are much more complex than the ones given here. These are meant to be simplified models of types of positions being taken in the current debate. It is obvious that those who believe that death means the irreversible loss of the capacity for bodily integration (3) or the irreversible loss of consciousness (4) have no reservations about pronouncing death when the heart and lungs have ceased to function. This is because they are willing to use loss of heart and lung activity as shortcut criteria for death, believing that once heart and lungs have stopped, the brain or neocortex will necessarily stop as well.

Source: Robert M. Veatch, *Death, Dying and the Biological Revolution* (New Haven: Yale University Press, 1976), p. 53.

rather than to define what is *right*. The biological aspects of medicine are not ambiguous in describing and predicting the processes of life and death, but by themselves they contribute very little to our moral decisions, decisions made necessary by increasing scientific knowledge. Medicine could effect a transplant in the Bill Samuels case, but it could not tell us if it was *right* to do so.

All thinking people are concerned about the "right" and "wrong" uses of our unprecedented knowledge and power. For help in finding our own answers to these moral questions, we cannot turn to medicine itself, but rather to the traditional repositories of moral insight in our society—law, philosophy, and theology.

The legal community needs a clear and acceptable definition of death because it must be prepared to act in a variety of ways upon the death of an individual. A declaration of death sets into motion a series of events that alter the legal status of the dead person and his or her survivors. Determinations must be made about transmission of wealth and property, insurance and taxes, and the marital status of the remaining spouse, to name a few. The body of the deceased itself becomes the property of the family, and that brings responsibilities for the family.

Despite these needs and the legal preference for precision, the legal community cannot by itself develop and enforce its own definition of death. However, in 1975 the American Bar Association adopted a resolution recommending the brain death definition: "For all legal purposes a human body with irreversible cessation of total brain function according to usual and customary standards of medical practice shall be considered dead." At the same time, the cardiopulmonary definition of death is still used actively in the legal world. The laws of some states include both definitions in the same law regarding the definition of death, without distinguishing which is to take precedence. Still other states have held to the heart death definition exclusively, and others refer only to brain death. Thus, we can find ourselves in the position of saying that at a given moment a particular patient may be legally alive in one state and legally dead in another! In states that honor both definitions of death, the patient may be declared alive by one doctor and dead by another in the same case. The law, then, is not itself sufficient. Rather, it constitutes an instrument for the enforcement of convictions we hold.

PHILOSOPHY: HUMAN BEING, HUMAN THING

As you read this book, you have size, weight, density, and color. In some sense you are an arrangement of elements—atoms and molecules, solids and fluids. You share many characteristics with things, and yet it is automatic for you to think of yourself not as a thing, but as a human being.

Now think of Bill Samuels, whom we discussed at the beginning of this chapter—heart and kidneys functioning, lungs functioning with the assistance of a respirator but with a "dead" brain. In that condition was Bill a thing or a human being? For many, the answer to this question is not yet clear.

When artificial support was withdrawn from Bill Samuels, three other very sick patients were waiting for transplantation of his heart and kidneys. In this case, the recipients were found quickly. What if they had not been found so easily? Suppose it had taken several weeks or several months to locate recipients whose tissues matched Bill Samuels's? Do you think it would have been legitimate to keep Bill on the respirator throughout that search, in order to keep his heart and kidneys "fresh"? The following excerpts from a British journal contain a fascinating exchange between Lord Smith of Marlow, president of the Royal Society of Medicine, and Michael Lockwood, a philosopher at Oxford University. Lord Smith considers the question, Should a dying person be put on a respirator solely to preserve his or her organs for transplantation to waiting recipients?

Some have asked the question—Does this not merely exchange one ethical dilemma for another, for having identified 'brain-death' is it right to continue artificial support if the object cannot any longer be to help the patient and can only be to preserve organs for possible transplantation? The answer must surely be that a doctor does not have the same responsibility towards a dead body as he does towards a live patient, and that to preserve artificially the organs of a recently dead patient for the possible advantage of other live patients is entirely right and cannot be criticised so long as a proper regard is paid to the sensitivities and feelings of relatives. A much more difficult question to answer arises when a patient terminally ill with a grossly inoperable cerebral tumour stops breathing. Now—knowing that it cannot help the patient who is beyond help, though still alive, is it ehtical to put the patient on a respirator solely in order to preserve organs for transplantation? If the views of the patient and relatives are known, there is no real difficulty, but supposing the views are not known, what then?[2]

Michael Lockwood responds:

I turn, finally, to Lord Smith's remarks concerning the maintenance of body function, in the now or soon to be brain dead, solely for the purpose of providing a supply of transplantable organs. There is, without doubt, something ghoulish in this conception; and it is this feeling, perhaps, that prompts Lord Smith to think that there is an ethical problem here. But provided it is a question of the prolongation merely of body function, and not, say, suffering, can there, on reflection, be any rational objection to this practice? Any lingering sense that there is can only, I should have thought, be evidence of doctors (and the public at large) having failed

2. Lord Smith of Marlow, "Closing Remarks on Ethical Problems in Surgical Practice," *Journal of Medical Ethics* 6 (June 1980): 79.

to accept with their hearts what they have already accepted with their heads: namely that a brain dead patient is, after all, dead. The heart may be beating, and the lungs respiring, but the body is nevertheless a corpse, not a living human being. In the end, the surgeon who has lost a patient might even find solace in the thought that his efforts have not been entirely in vain—if the preservation of body function, by his skill, can serve to enhance or even save the lives of others.

. . . Suffice it to say that it is very reassuring for the layman to find, amongst surgeons, such sensitivity to the ethical implications of their work. With the advance in surgical science, one finds that what once were questions largely for philosophical debate, turn with bewildering rapidity into matters of widespread public concern.[3]

Not all philosophers would agree with Lockwood's answer to Lord Smith's question. Some offer possible justifications for continuing to treat patients who have suffered brain death. They argue that ambiguous biological data make it risky to draw lines arbitrarily between life and death by creating "definitions." They argue also that if patients are to be treated as human beings up through the ends of their lives, then artificial life-support systems ought not to be used to maintain the patient's body after brain death has occurred. In other words, we should not allow medical technology to be used to turn a human being into a thing under any circumstances. The temptation to do this for a "good" reason, such as to gain organs for transplantation, is too great.

THEOLOGY: BODY AND SOUL

Before we had the capacity to maintain breathing artificially by machine, and in other ways to postpone death, the "moment" of death was regarded as occurring with the last breath. One way to say a person was dead was to say he or she had "expired," a word rooted in the same word from which the English language derives "spirit," "inspire," and "respiration."

In Jewish and Christian belief and symbolism, bodily respiration was linked to the "breath of life." From one of the Genesis stories of creation in which God breathed the breath of life into the human creature made from the dust of the earth, breathing and breath were associated with the divine aspect of each human being. Therefore, the cessation of breathing was considered the "moment" of death. In medieval Christian art the soul is sometimes depicted escaping out of the body with the last breath.

While most modern people no longer maintain such a direct connection between a physiological phenomenon—breathing or its cessation—and spiritual beliefs, modern medical developments such as respirators gener-

3. Michael Lockwood, "Ethical Dilemmas in Surgery: Some Philosophical Reflections," *Journal of Medical Ethics* 6 (June 1980): 82–84.

ate intriguing questions for religious believers and nonbelievers. In a modern, secular world where the majority of religious believers no longer profess a naive, tacit belief in a connection between natural phenomena, such as breathing, and spiritual values, there remains still a residual link between cessation of breathing and death. Three physicians recently traced the links among words such as "air, breath and spirit" in Hebrew, Greek, Sanskrit, Chinese, and languages of Africa and New Guinea.[4] The long-standing, universal connections between breathing and spiritual status are maintained even in a secularized world, they point out. They conclude: "The powerful linguistic ties between breath and spirit attest to an old human need to relate physiological and spiritual aspects of life. Our patients remind us that this need has not disappeared."

What happens to values, beliefs and symbols about the "moment" of death when respirators and other medical developments can maintain breathing mechanically and when breathing can be maintained after the brain is "dead"? In his lengthy history of death and dying, Philippe Aries[5] has pointed out that some recent liturgical changes made for Roman Catholics signal a change in modern religious belief and practice. He notes that the rite of Extreme Unction has been done away with, and in its place is an annointing of the sick. With there no longer being a "moment" of death beyond human intervention, the rite intended to be the last liturgical act performed for a believer has been replaced by a rite not limited to those near death, nor necessarily even terminally ill.

While this one particular example from Catholic liturgy indicates a shift in religious belief and values about the "moment" of death and its traditional link to cessation of breathing, medical developments raise other questions which do not produce such specific answers. What about the status of the human body? Is it merely a *receptacle* for the spirit? If breathing is maintained but the brain is "dead," is the person dead in a spiritual sense as well as a physiological sense? When *is* the "moment" of death? What other religious beliefs, symbols, or rites will have to be altered as a result of new medical knowledge and technologies? Will these developments enhance or detract from the way Jews and Christians regard the human body and its relationship to the "spirit"?

These questions are made even more urgent by medical developments in organ transplantation. Jews, for example, traditionally have held to specific beliefs and ritual practices regarding a corpse. But transplanting an organ from one person whose breathing is maintained artificially but whose brain is "dead" could be regarded as a new form of charity among

---

4. Joachim S. Gravenstein, Santosh Kalhan, and Nikolas G. Balamoutsos, "Of Breath and Spirits," *Journal of the American Medical Association* 246 (1981): 1091–92.

5. Philippe Aries, *The Hour of Our Death* (New York: Alfred A. Knopf, 1981).

some Christians. In fact, this has been the case. Some individual Christians regard participating in organ donation programs as giving a gift, perhaps an eye, kidneys or heart and lungs, to another person at the time of the donor's death. Other believers, such as Jews and some Christians with special regard for the human body and specific assumptions about a corpse or person near death, could consider this possibility with horror.

ORGAN TRANSPLANTATION AND DETERMINING DEATH

Until the late 1960s medical scientists could only dream of the possibility of transferring a heart from a patient like Bill Samuels to a patient who could not live without it. When medicine crossed the threshold into the era of successful transplantation, society's need for ethical and legal definitions was intensified.

The practice of transferring body substances from one person to another for the benefit of the recipient is not new. Blood transfusions between persons whose blood types match has been going on since the 1930s, but the first successful organ transplants in humans did not occur until December 1967, when Dr. Christiaan Barnard performed a successful heart transplant. By the beginning of the 1980s, disillusionment with heart transplantation had set in because of the high mortality rate and the extreme cost of the surgical procedure and postoperative care. Nevertheless, experimentation continues in transplantation of the heart, the heart together with the lungs, and the kidneys. Advances are being made every year, and questions about when to declare death remain crucial.

Let us return again to the case of Bill Samuels. His brain seemed to be dead, and yet his respiration was being maintained artificially. The obvious question is whether under these circumstances the man was dead or alive. If such a patient is declared formally to be alive, then he must be treated as a patient in critical condition, with all the rights of a living person. If he is formally declared to be dead, then he is merely a corpse with two vital functions being maintained artificially. Under these conditions health care directed to saving his life may cease, and the society may legitimately begin the emotional and legal changes that normally follow death. The scenario may take some new turns if the dying person is to be regarded as a potential donor of lifesaving organs. Think about this from the viewpoint of (1) a doctor whose reflex is to save life where possible, and (2) from the viewpoint of another patient whose heart or kidneys are diseased.

Once death has been pronounced, by whatever criteria, there is a need to move quickly. Complicated surgery must begin on both the deceased and the organ recipient(s). At some point in the treatment of a brain-dead patient, it is only natural that the doctor and the potential recipient begin to think in terms of preserving the life of the patient's heart or kidneys. This concern can be acted upon only when there is absolutely no possibility that the life of the whole patient can be preserved. We have achieved something approaching a consensus about this matter and about the designation of brain death as the proper criterion for a formal declaration of death. However, many ambiguities remain in how precisely to formulate what brain death *is,* that is, which parts of the brain must be dead and how they can be known to be dead.

The available consensus is now finding its way into law, as we have said. In 1968 Kansas became the first state to pass laws relevant to these questions. One permitted the procurement of organs specifically for transplantation and another gave legal status to brain death. By now, about half of the states have adopted some form of brain death definition. In all states there now is a Uniform Anatomical Gift Act. In 1981, a Uniform Determination of Death Act was proposed for consideration by state legislatures.

As events actually unfolded in the 1960s and 1970s, organ transplantation and brain death definitions became linked. Because the first state statute, in Kansas, to incorporate brain death as a criterion for determining death also included new laws for organ transplantation, there was some criticism that a new definition of death had been created to supply organs for the then fledgling medical procedures for organ transplantation. We believe medical developments would have forced the issue of determining death upon us anyway.

THE UNIFORM ANATOMICAL GIFT ACT

The Anatomical Gift! That is one of those terms that seems ordinary at first, and then absolutely stunning upon reflection. The Uniform Anatomical Gift Act (UAGA) was proposed by the National Conference of Commissioners on Uniform State Laws in its final form in July 1968. The act deliberately avoided the problem of defining death because its authors feared that the complicated nature of that discussion might delay passage of UAGA. As it turned out, passage was swift. By 1972 all fifty states had adopted statutes, based on the UAGA proposal, to set rules by which essential organs could be taken from cadavers for research or from recently deceased persons for research or transplantation. Excerpts from the UAGA are reprinted in the article by Alexander Capron and Leon Kass at the end of this chapter.

As the case of Bill Samuels illustrated, the UAGA (as adopted in all states) is built on the assumption that the donor leaves explicit instructions for his or her body, or certain parts of it, to be used for research or transplantation at death. The donor fills out a card, which is carried at all times, indicating the specific choice he or she has made. (By contrast, some European donor statutes are built on the opposite assumption; all persons are potential donors at death *unless* they carry a card indicating specifically they do *not* wish to be a donor.) The UAGA is specific about how permission is to be secured for a donation. A donor card (see figure 3), or legal will, or some other recognized record must be filled out by the

---

UNIFORM DONOR CARD

OF_____

Print or type name of donor

In the hope that I may help others, I hereby make this anatomical gift, if medically acceptable, to take effect upon my death. The words and marks below indicate my desires.

I give: (a) _____ any needed organs or parts

   (b) _____ only the following organs or parts

_____

Specify the organ(s) or part(s)

for the purposes of transplantation, therapy, medical research or education;

   (c) _____ my body for anatomical study if needed.

Limitations or
special wishes, if any :_____

08-21-81 100M/82

Signed by the donor and the following two witnesses in the presence of each other:

_____   _____
Signature of Donor   Date of Birth of Donor

_____   _____
Date Signed   City & State

_____   _____
Witness   Witness

This is a legal document under the Uniform Anatomical Gift Act or similar laws.

For further information consult your physician or

National Kidney Foundation, Inc.
2 Park Avenue, New York, N.Y. 10016

donor and witnessed before he or she loses the ability to make decisions. In the absence of such a document, the family still may make donations of the body or organs of the deceased. This is in keeping with the fact that the body becomes property of the next of kin. The UAGA is specific in requiring that the time of death be certified by a doctor (in some states, two doctors). Further, the doctor who attends the donor at death may not participate in the removal or transplantation of organs.

THE "UNIFORM DETERMINATION OF DEATH"

In 1981, the President's Commission for the Study of Ethical Problems in Medicine and Biomedical and Behavioral Research recommended a uniform determination of death and proposed it be adopted in all states. The model statute proposed is simple and may be quoted in its entirety:

An individual who has sustained either (1) irreversible cessation of circulatory and respiratory functions, or (2) irreversible cessation of all functions of the entire brain, including the brain stem, is dead. A determination of death must be made in accordance with accepted medical standards.[6]

This proposal has several key features. First, it uses a whole-brain criterion for determining death and rejects cessation of only the "higher" functions. Second, it allows for using *either* cessation of circulatory and respiratory functions *or* a brain death criterion. Third, it leaves the procedure of how cessation of brain activity is to be measured to "accepted medical standards." The first feature is considered the more conservative and less controversial choice. The second feature takes into account that most declarations of death still will be made adequately according to traditional detection of cessation of heartbeat and breathing. The third feature leaves undefined the procedures to measure brain activity because new medical technologies are evolving.

The acceptance, rejection, or changes that might be made in this proposed statute is a topic of current deliberation. As we have attempted to indicate, such deliberation is important for at least two reasons:

1. The concepts embedded in such statutes have practical ramifications:
   a. Who is dead or who is alive in the eyes of the law?
   b. How are the rights of persons caught "between" definitions to be protected?

6. Minutes of Meeting XI of the President's Commission for the Study of Ethical Problems in Medicine and Biomedical and Behavioral Research, published by the commission on August 28, 1981, p. 3.

2. Such concepts, especially when made law, translate our values into concrete guides which permit or prohibit human behavior:
   a. Does this proposed statute convey the value we place on human life?
   b. What effect does it have on the way we regard death and treat the dead?

The current public debate surrounding this proposed statute—public hearings, the wording of the law actually proposed in your state, and the likely court cases that will result—all are part of the process by which an open, democratic society makes its choices. Either as an individual or as a member of a professional or special interest organization, you have many points at which you can participate in the deliberation and resolution of a uniform determination of death.

SELECTED READINGS
A Hierarchy of Rules Defining Death[7]

A person will be considered dead if in the announced opinion of a physician, based on ordinary standards of medical practice, he has experienced an irreversible cessation of spontaneous respiratory and circulatory functions. In the event that artificial means of support preclude a determination that these functions have ceased, a person will be considered dead if in the announced opinion of a physician, based on ordinary standards of medical practice, he has experienced an irreversible cessation of spontaneous brain functions. Death will have occurred at the time when the relevant functions ceased.

First, the proposal speaks in terms of the *death* of a *person*. The determination that a person has died is to be based on an evaluation of certain vital bodily functions, the permanent absence of which indicates that he is no longer a living human being. By concentrating on the death of a human being as a whole, the statute rightly disregards the fact that some cells or organs may continue to "live" after this point, just as others may have ceased functioning long before the determination of death. This statute would leave for resolution by other means the question of when the absence or deterioration of certain capacities, such as the ability to communicate, or functions, such as the cerebral, indicates that a person may or should be allowed to die without further medical intervention.

Second, the proposed legislation is predicated upon the single phenomenon of death. Moreover, it applies uniformly to all persons, by specifying the circumstances under which each of the standards is to be used rather than leaving this to the unguided discretion of physicians. Unlike the Kansas law, the model statute

---

7. Excerpts from Alexander Capron and Leon Kass, "A Statutory Definition of the Standards for Determining Human Death: An Appraisal and a Proposal," *University of Pennsylvania Law Review* 121 (November 1972): 87–88 (copyright by *University of Pennsylvania Law Review*).

does not leave to arbitrary decision a choice between two apparently equal yet different "alternative definitions of death." Rather, its second standard is applicable only when "artificial means of support preclude" use of the first. It does not establish a separate kind of death, called "brain death." In other words, the proposed law would provide two standards gauged by different functions, for measuring different manifestations of the same phenomenon. If cardiac and pulmonary functions have ceased, brain functions cannot continue; if there is no brain activity and respiration has to be maintained artificially, the same state (i.e., death) exists. Some people might prefer a single standard, one based either on cardiopulmonary or brain functions. This would have the advantage of removing the last trace of the "two deaths" image, which any reference to alternative standards may still leave. Respiratory and circulatory indicators, once the only touchstone, are no longer adequate in some situations. It would be possible, however, to adopt the alternative, namely that death is *always* to be established by assessing spontaneous brain functions. Reliance only on brain activity, however, would represent a sharp and unnecessary break with tradition. Departing from continuity with tradition is not only theoretically unfortunate in that it violates another principle of good legislation suggested previously, but also practically very difficult, since most physicians customarily employ cardiopulmonary tests for death and would be slow to change, especially when the old tests are easier to perform, more accessible and acceptable to the lay public, and perfectly adequate for determining death in most instances.

Finally, by adopting standards for death in terms of the cessation of certain vital bodily functions but not in terms of the specific criteria or tests by which these functions are to be measured, the statute does not prevent physicians from adapting their procedures to changes in medical technology.

A basic substantive issue remains: what are the merits of the proposed standards? For ordinary situations, the appropriateness of the traditional standard, "an irreversible cessation of spontaneous respiratory and circulatory functions," does not require elaboration. Indeed, examination by a physician may be more a formal than a real requirement in determining that most people have died. In addition to any obvious injuries, elementary signs of death such as absence of heartbeat and breathing, cold skin, fixed pupils, and so forth, are usually sufficient to indicate even to a layman that the accident victim, the elderly person who passes away quietly in the night, or the patient stricken with a sudden infarct has died. The difficulties arise when modern medicine intervenes to sustain a patient's respiration and circulation. As we noted in discussing the Harvard Committee's conclusions, the indicators of brain damage appear reliable, in that studies have shown that patients who fit the Harvard criteria have suffered such extensive damage that they do not recover. Of course, the task of the neurosurgeon or physician is simplified in the common case where an accident victim has suffered such gross, apparent injuries to the head that it is not necessary to apply the Harvard criteria in order to establish cessation of brain functioning.

The statutory standard, "irreversible cessation of spontaneous brain functions," is intended to encompass both higher brain activities and those of the brainstem.

There must, of course, also be no spontaneous respiration; the second standard is applied only when breathing is being artificially maintained. The major emphasis placed on brain functioning, although generally consistent with the common view of what makes man distinctive as a living creature, brings to the fore a basic issue: What aspects of brain function should be decisive? The question has been re-framed by some clinicians in light of their experience with patients who have undergone what they term "neocortical death" (that is, complete destruction of higher brain capacity, demonstrated by a flat E.E.G.). "Once neocortical death has been unequivocally established and the possibility of any recovery of con-sciousness and intellectual activity [is] thereby excluded, . . . although [the] pa-tient breathes spontaneously, is he or she alive?" While patients with irreversible brain damage from cardiac arrest seldom survive more than a few days, cases have recently been reported of survival for up to two and one-quarter years. Nevertheless, though existence in this state falls far short of a full human life, the very fact of spontaneous respiration, as well as coordinated movements and reflex activities at the brainstem and spinal cord levels, would exclude these patients from the scope of the statutory standards. The condition of "neocortical death" may well be a proper justification for interrupting all forms of treatment and allowing these patients to die, but this moral and legal problem cannot and should not be settled by "defining" these people "dead."

The legislation suggested here departs from the Kansas statute in its basic approach to the problem of "defining" death: the proposed statute does not set about to establish a special category of "brain death" to be used by transplanters. Further, there are a number of particular points of difference between them. For example, the proposed statute does not speak of persons being "medically and legally dead," thus avoiding redundancy and, more importantly, the mistaken implication that that "medical" and "legal" definitions could differ. Also, the proposed legislation does not include the provision that "death is to be pro-nounced before" the machine is turned off or any organs removed. Such a *modus operandi*, which was incorporated by Kansas from the Harvard Committee's report, may be advisable for physicians on public relations grounds, but it has no place in a statute "defining" death. The proposed statute already provides that "Death will have occurred at the time when the relevant functions ceased." If supportive aids, or organs, are withdrawn after this time, such acts cannot be implicated as having caused death. The manner in which, or exact time at which, the physician should articulate his finding is a matter best left to the exigencies of the situation, to local medical customs or hospital rules, or to statutes on the procedures for certifying death or on transplantation if the latter is the procedure which raises the greatest concern of medical impropriety. The real safeguard against doctors killing patients is not to be found in a statute "defining" death. Rather, it inheres in physicians' ethical and religious beliefs, which are also embodied in the fundamental professional ethic of *primum non nocere* and are reinforced by homicide and "wrongful death" laws and the rules governing medi-cal negligence applicable in license revocation proceedings or in private actions for damages.

The proposed statute shares with the Kansas legislation two features of which Professor Kennedy is critical. First, it does not require that two physicians participate in determining death, as recommended by most groups which set forth suggestions about transplatation. The reasons for the absence of such a provision should be obvious. Since the statute deals with death in general and not with death in relation to transplantation, there is no reason for it to establish a general rule which is required only in that unusual situation. If particular dangers lurk in the transplantation setting, they should be dealt with in legislation on that subject, such as the Uniform Anatomical Gift Act. If all current means of determining "irreversible cessation of spontaneous brain functions" are inherently so questionable that they should be double-checked by a second (or third, fourth, etc.) physician to be trustworthy, or if a certain means of measuring brain function requires as a technical matter the cooperation of two, or twenty, physicians, then the participation of the requisite number of experts would be part of the "ordinary standards of medical practice" that circumscribe the proper, non-negligent use of such procedures. It would be unfortunate, however, to introduce such a requirement into legislation which sets forth the general standards for determining who is dead, especially when it is done in such a way as to differentiate between one standard and another.

Kennedy's second objection, that a death statute ought to provide "for the separation and insulation of the physician (or physicians) attending the patient donor and certifying death, from the recipient of any organ that may be salvaged from the cadaver," is likewise unnecessary. As was noted previously, language that relates only to transplantation has no place in a statute on the determination of death.

Changes in medical knowledge and procedures have created an apparent need for a clear and acceptable revision of the standards for determining that a person has died. Some commentators have argued that the formulation of such standards should be left to physicians. The reasons for rejecting this argument seem compelling: the "definition of death" is not merely a matter for technical expertise, the uncertainty of the present law is unhealthy for society and physicians alike, there is a great potential for mischief and harm through the possibility of conflict between the standards applied by some physicians and those assumed to be applicable by the community at large and its legal system, and patients and their relatives are made uneasy by physicians apparently being free to shift around the meaning of death without any societal guidance. Accordingly, we conclude the public has a legitimate role to play in the formulation and adoption of such standards. This article has proposed a model statute which bases a determination of death primarily on the traditional standard of final respiratory and circulatory cessation; where the artificial maintenance of these functions precludes the use of such a standard, the statute authorizes that death be determined on the basis of irreversible cessation of spontaneous brain functions. We believe the legislation proposed would dispel public confusion and concern and protect physicians and patients, while avoiding the creation of "two types of death," for which the statute on this subject first adopted in Kansas has been justly criticized. The proposal is offered not as the ultimate solution to the problem, but as a catalyst for what we hope will be a robust and well-informed public debate over a new "definition." Finally, the proposed statute leaves for future resolution the even more difficult problems concerning the conditions and procedures under which a decision may be reached to cease treating a terminal patient who does not meet the standards set forth in the statutory "definition of death."

Limiting the Alternatives of Individual Choice[8]

What if Aunt Bertha says she knows Uncle Charlie's brain is completely destroyed and his heart is not beating and his lungs are not functioning, but she still thinks there is hope—she still thinks of him as her loving husband and does not want death pronounced for a few more days? Worse yet, what if a grown son who has long since abandoned his senile, mentally ill, and institutionalized father decides that his father's life has lost whatever makes it essentially human and chooses to have him called dead even though his heart, lungs, and brain continue to function? Clearly society cannot permit every individual to choose literally any concept of death. For the same reason, the shortsighted acceptance of death as meaning whatever physicians choose for it to mean is wrong. A physician agreeing with either Aunt Bertha or the coldhearted son should certainly be challenged by society and its judicial system.

There must, then, be limits on individual freedom. At this moment in history the reasonable choices for a concept of death are those focusing on respiration and circulation, on the body's integrating capacities, and on consciousness and related social interactions. Allowing individual choice among these viable alternatives, but not beyond them, may be the only way out of this social policy impasse.

To develop model legislation, we can begin with the Capron-Kass statutory proposal and make several changes to avoid the problems we have discussed. First, a cerebral locus for determining if a person is dead can be incorporated by simply changing the word *brain* to the narrower *cerebral*. Second, it seems to me a reasonable safeguard to insist, in general terms appropriate for a statutory definition, that there be no significant conflict of interest. Finally, wording should be added to permit freedom of choice within reasonable limits. These changes would create the following statute specifying the standards for determining that a person has died:

A person will be considered dead if in the announced opinion of a physician, based on ordinary standards of medical practice, he has experienced an irreversible cessation of spontaneous respiratory and circulatory functions. In the event that artificial means of support preclude a determination that these functions have ceased, a person will be considered dead if in the announced opinion of a physician, based on ordinary standards of medical practice, he has experienced an irreversible cessation of spontaneous cerebral functions. Death will have occurred at the time when the relevant functions ceased. It is

8. Excerpts from Robert Veatch, *Death, Dying and the Biological Revolution* (New Haven: Yale University Press, 1976), pp. 75–76.

provided, however, that no person shall be considered dead even with the announced opinion of a physician solely on the basis of an irreversible cessation of spontaneous cerebral functions if he, while competent to make such a decision, has explicitly rejected the use of this standard or, if he has not expressed himself on the matter while competent, his legal guardian or next of kin explicitly expresses such rejection.

It is further provided that no physician shall pronounce the death of any individual in any case where there is significant conflict of interest with his obligation to serve the patient (including commitment to any other patients, research, or teaching programs which might directly benefit from pronouncing the patient dead).

Death Watch[9]

It may not seem the most appropriate topic for a summer's morning, but a public body with the cumbersome title, the President's Commission for the Study of Ethical Problems in Medicine and Biomedical and Behavioral Research, is getting ready to present President Reagan this fall with a report on the definition of death. This is neither so depressing nor so arcane an event as it may sound.

The commission was established by statute to report on a whole range of medical-ethical questions and the problem of defining death certainly deserves its place on the list. In recent years the courts and the newspapers have been peppered with stories about how advancing medical technology is making it ever harder to distinguish between the living and the dead, the treatable and the hopeless. This report offers a way to begin quieting the problem.

The issue is as deep as the old, near-universal human fear of waking up in a coffin. In recent years it has acquired newly macabre forms. Mechanical respirators are making it possible to sustain a body's breathing well past its natural point of expiration. This enables people to begin worrying about whether the plug will get pulled on a human who otherwise would have lived to recover some day.

The improving technology of organ transplants makes the fear more vivid: Someone will now have a real reason to pull that plug. So when experts start talking about how we should no longer consider a person alive just because he's breathing, and how we should instead start using brain-function criteria as a way of determining death, the layman suspects something fishy is going on.

The commission has come up with a suggested standard: We should consider people dead either according to the traditional criteria of whether their breathing and circulation have irreversibly stopped or—if mechanical intervention makes it impossible to tell this—according to whether all their brain functions have irreversibly ceased. This includes the brain-stem impulses that make breathing possible; when these are irrevocably gone, the breathing induced by a mechanical respirator is only an imitation of life.

This formula is brief but represents a good number of decisions made. It is to be administered according to an elaborate set of clinical tests and safeguards. It

9. Editorial from the *Wall Street Journal*, August 25, 1981. Reprinted by permission of the *Wall Street Journal*, © Dow Jones & Co., Inc., 1981. All Rights Reserved.

rejects one popular idea proposed to the commission, the concept that people should be considered dead when their higher brain functions or personalities are gone. It explicitly does not apply to the coma of a Karen Anne Quinlan, who breathes without a respirator. The new standard's emphasis on the whole brain and on irreversibility is meant to separate the definition of death from the question of abortion or of euthanasia for the dying, rather than to open the door to these topics.

The commission would like the states to adopt this standard in place of the varying and confusing definitions now in place. There is enough need for uniformity in the area so that they should do so. The approaches to and away from life are going to be littered for years to come by the new questions that technology raises. But we should cope where we can; and this is one piece of the dilemma that we should, for the moment, try to lay to rest.

ANNOTATED BIBLIOGRAPHY
Books and Articles

Black, Peter M. "Brain Death." *New England Journal of Medicine* 299 (1978): 338–44, 393–401. A general and synoptic presentation of the nature and significance of current brain death issues by a physician and philosopher. Emphasizes medically related issues.

Byrne, Paul A., et al. "Brain Death—An Opposing Viewpoint." *Journal of the American Medical Association* 242 (1979): 1985–90. The meaning of the word "death" is discussed, and qualms are registered about some forms of "brain death" and some policies of organ procurement.

Engelhardt, H. Tristram. "Definition of Death: Where to Draw the Lines and Why." In *Death and Decision,* ed. Ernan McMullin. Boulder, Colo.: Westview Press, 1978. Pp. 15–34. A conceptual more than medical analysis, in which the decisional nature of defining death and the purposes surrounding such definitions are explored. The article emphasizes philosophical rather than medical issues. (Other articles in this same volume are also quite helpful.)

Institute of Society, Ethics, and the Life Sciences, Task Force on Death and Dying. "Refinements in Criteria for the Determination of Death." *Journal of the American Medical Association* 221 (1972): 48–53. An interdisciplinary group of distinguished humanists and scientists collaborated to produce this policy-oriented document.

Anthologies

Beauchamp, Tom L., and Seymour Perlin, eds. *Ethical Issues in Death and Dying.* Englewood Cliffs, N.J.: Prentice-Hall, 1978. Chaps. 1 and 3. Chapter 1 contains an outstanding group of essays on medical, social, and philosophical topics surrounding the definition of death. Chapter 3 focuses on patients' rights in the dying circumstance.

Korein, Julius, ed. "Brain Death: Interrelated Medical and Social Issues." *Annals of the New York Academy of Sciences* 315 (1978): 1–454. A special issue that is distinctly medically oriented, yet contains a series of very useful articles on the philosophical, ethical, and legal problems of brain death.

Articles from the *Encyclopedia of Bioethics*

Death
  I. Anthropological Perspective *David Landy*
 II. Eastern Thought *Frank E. Reynolds*
III. Western Philosophical Thought *James Gutmann*
 IV. Western Religious Thought
     1. Death in Biblical Thought *Lloyd Bailey*
     2. Post-Biblical Jewish Tradition *Seymour Siegel*
     3. Post-Biblical Christian Thought *Milton McC. Gatch*
     4. Ars Moriendi *Brian P. Copenhaver*
  V. Death in the Western World *Talcott Parsons*
Attitudes toward Death *Richard A. Kalish*
Definition and Determination of Death
  I. Criteria for Death *Gaetano F. Molinari*
 II. Legal Aspects of Pronouncing Death *Alexander Morgan Capron*
III. Philosophical and Theological Foundations *Dallas M. High*

Literature

Poe, Edgar Allan. "The Facts in the Case of M. Valdemar." In *Introduction to Poe*, ed. E. W. Carlson. Glenview, Ill.: Scott, Foresman and Co., 1967. Poe's short story describes an experiment in which M. Valdemar is hypnotized at the point of death. When they try to awaken him, he cries "For God's Sake!—quick!—quick!—put me to sleep—or, quick! waken!—quick!—*I say to you that I am dead!*" Although a short story unique to Poe's imagination, it captures the unease many sense when a person is dead by one "definition" but not by another.

5

INFORMED CONSENT: HOW MUCH DO YOU HAVE TO KNOW?

By exposure to a sick co-worker, John Marx contracted a severe case of hepatitis. When Marx was admitted to the hospital Dr. Nancy Green studied his medical history and discovered that he was habituated to phenobarbital. He had started taking the drug two years previously as a sedative, and by this time was taking six tablets daily. This presented a problem. Ordinarily, Dr. Green might not have considered trying to deal with the phenobarbital problem while treating another illness; in the case of Mr. Marx she felt that she had to withdraw the phenobarbital in order to prevent a rapid and dangerous buildup of the drug in Mr. Marx's blood. The liver of a hepatitis patient does not cleanse the bloodstream efficiently. Besides, Dr. Green could find no present indication of a medical need for phenobarbital.

Dr. Green instructed the pharmacy to prepare pills containing decreasing amounts of phenobarbital and increasing amounts of an inert substance. She prescribed the pills so that Mr. Marx believed that he was receiving his accustomed dosage of phenobarbital. In truth, he was being withdrawn from the drug over a period of days without his knowledge. Dr. Green monitored Mr. Marx's blood chemistry each day to confirm that phenobarbital levels were becoming lower. In spite of this precaution, on the fourth hospital day Mr. Marx had an epileptic seizure, a known potential complication of barbiturate withdrawal. During the seizure Mr. Marx fell from his bed and broke his arm.

Mr. Marx eventually brought suit against Dr. Green for damage resulting from Dr. Green's failure to secure informed consent from her patient for the treatment she had decided was prudent and medically indicated. Marx's attorney argued that a detoxification program was active therapy. Furthermore, the doctrine of informed consent was argued to be applicable because convulsions are a known possible risk of phenobarbital withdrawal, and Mr. Marx was not informed of the nature of his treatment or its possible risks.

A Question to Consider

Why, in fact, did Dr. Green withhold information from her patient? Mr. Marx and his attorneys asserted that she had done so because she felt that Mr. Marx would object strenuously and might refuse the prescribed regimen if he knew that he was being taken off phenobarbital. Dr. Green denied that this was the reason. The doctor and her attorneys argued that in his addicted state, John Marx was in no condition to make an informed, voluntary, and prudent judgment about his own treatment. Dr. Green's attorneys invoked *"therapeutic privilege,"* under which it is legal to withhold information if the doctor believes that disclosing the information might seriously harm the patient.

A CONFLICT OF DUTIES

This case illustrates a moral dilemma that is acutely felt by patients and health care practitioners. The dilemma is a choice between two honored duties: telling the truth and caring for the patient when care includes not telling the complete truth. In traditional literature about medical ethics, law, and moral theology and philosophy, this dilemma often has been described as a choice between truth-telling and invoking therapeutic privilege to conceal information. The phrase "truth-telling" is self-explanatory, and in the health care context it simply means that the doctor is obliged to tell his or her patient the truth. On the other hand, a therapeutic privilege justifies a doctor in *withholding* information or even *lying* when in his or her medical professional judgment serious harm would be caused to a patient by a disclosure. In situations when telling the truth may be bad practice, it is argued that the doctrine of therapeutic privilege may be validly invoked by the physician.

THE NEW SITUATION

A variety of factors have presented a new twist on the classical dilemma between telling the truth and withholding or altering the truth. Because we daily live with many of these factors, a brief list will suffice to summarize the new situations:

1. Medical information is increasingly sophisticated, and special efforts are required to convey information to patients.
2. Diagnostic procedures provide information to health care specialists sometimes long before there are symptoms and before the patient has any awareness of future medical problems.
3. Specialization by doctors and other health care practitioners can result in a patient dealing with a team of specialists, with whom it is difficult, if not impossible, to develop a relationship. In those cases the practi-

tioner cannot gauge intelligently the best level of information to provide to the patient and it is difficult for the patient to feel comfortable in seeking reliable information.

4. We live in an era of litigation, when misunderstandings routinely are brought to a court for settlement.

5. Consumerism, in which the recipient of goods or services attempts to seek information in order to make more informed decisions, has spread to health care.

6. Authority, especially the paternalism that has characterized the traditional doctor-patient relationship, is under more frequent challenge.

7. In recent years, the Western ideal of autonomy has become more clearly defined as courts and legislatures and other institutions have become more specific about self-determination and the "rights" of individuals.

8. Publicity about abuses by some medical researchers has been extensive.

9. In law, therapeutic privilege is strict and narrow. But in the practice of medicine it is highly valued as central to the "art" of medicine and the physician's discretionary use of information.

Whether one views these as good or bad developments, they are undeniably characteristics of our times and greatly influence the relationship between the patient and the health care professional. The crux of this contemporary dilemma seems to be in the exchange of information from professional to patient. How much information is a doctor *obligated* to give to a patient? How much information does a patient have a *"right"* to *know?* What happens to "therapeutic privilege" in this new era? How much information is needed for a patient to give an "informed consent"? What kind of information may be hazardous to the patient's health and what is the hazard?

These factors are illustrated in the kinds of contemporary situations similar to that of John Marx. The following story of Marie Bell is another example that shows the ways these factors emerge today.

AT HER CALIFORNIA HOME, MARIE BELL WAS LIVING ALONE FOR THE FIRST TIME IN MANY years. After twenty years as a wife and mother she was widowed and her children had moved away to school and work. Still, she had a circle of old friends and she felt that she might have made reasonable adjustment to her new station in life if it had not been for the headaches. Mrs. Bell's doctor and his office staff dreaded her visits, which were frequent. Mrs. Bell was cross and impatient with the staff and was extremely demanding both in the office and on the phone. After putting her in the hospital for a brief diagnostic routine, the doctor told Marie that she had hypertension. He discharged her from the hospital and prescribed her medication.

Marie insisted that the doctor had not explained fully the reasons for prescribing the medication, and she asked questions repeatedly about the side effects of the medicine. She complained that the doctor did not spend enough time with her in the office. She demanded precise details regarding his credentials and implied that he had had insufficient experience in treating hypertension. She seemed determined to find some inconsistency in what she was told. The doctor was more than a little relieved when Mrs. Bell announced that she was moving to Connecticut to accept an executive position with the Connecticut Welfare Department.

The new job was one that carried great responsibility and public trust. Marie managed programs that cost the taxpayers ten million dollars a year. She was plagued by headaches and was anxious and irritable. In Connecticut she visited several physicians until she found one who she felt could assume responsibility for her treatment. This doctor routinely requested the medical records from her hospitalization in California.

When the records arrived a remarkable discovery was made. Her doctor in California had done a CT scan of Marie's head. When her new doctor in Connecticut interpreted this computer-enhanced X ray, he concluded that Marie was suffering from the early stages of Pick's Disease, a rare disease involving a gradual degeneration of brain tissue. The cause of Pick's Disease is unknown, and there is no treatment for it. At first the patient begins to lose recent memory and judgment. Later, there is a progressive loss of higher intellectual function. Eventually, the victim is reduced to a vegetative state leading to death.

The Connecticut doctor realized that Marie knew nothing of the CT scan. He strongly suspected that her nervousness and irritating patterns of behavior were early manifestations of the disease itself. Naturally, his first thought was to tell Marie about both the diagnosis and the prognosis. He reasoned that full knowledge of her condition might allow her to make important decisions while she was still capable of doing so. It also occurred to him that unless she was told, Marie might actually become a hazard to a large and expensive program affecting thousands of people. He was in the habit of telling the truth to his patients, and he disliked withholding any information because of the uncomfortable feeling of dishonesty that such withholding produced in him. Other considerations caused him to hesitate. At the very least, Marie would be emotionally demolished by the news. Already she exhibited signs of being vulnerable to depression. The possibility of her suicide crossed the doctor's mind. In the face of her inevitable barrage of questions, he knew he would be able to say absolutely nothing to offer hope.

He finally elected not to tell Marie about her illness. He reasoned that concealing this information was an act of kindness and that it would work in the best interests of the patient. Furthermore, because memory loss is fairly swift and pronounced in Pick's Disease, Marie probably would never even be hurt by the realization that she had been deceived. He decided to find an opportunity to suggest that she put her affairs in order, just as a matter of prudent personal management. Then he would continue treating her as if neither of them were aware of the diagnosis. He would not take it upon himself to mention anything to Mrs. Bell's employer.

A Question to Consider

Do you think that Marie Bell's doctor did the right thing in concealing from her the fact that she was suffering from the early stages of an incurable, fatal illness? Medical professionals and lay persons alike have been groping for clear guidelines to follow in their expectations and behavior with respect to medical information. Doctors are sure that sometimes it is better for the patient not to know the whole story. On the other hand, even when the doctor decides to communicate fully with a patient, it is more difficult to do so than ever before. The concepts and the language of modern medicine are complicated. It may be difficult for a doctor to communicate enough accurate information to a patient so that a patient can make insightful judgments about his or her own treatment without jeopardizing the patient's welfare.

There is, then, a widening gap between lay knowledge and professional knowledge in medicine. The average "consumer" has high expectations of doctors, nurses, and medical laboratory technicians. There is some evidence to suggest that movies, novels, and television dramas have led us to expect almost miraculous results from the efforts of these professionals. At the same time, consumers have become vaguely uneasy about the fact that they understand so little of what doctors are doing. There is a growing tendency for patients to "shop around" for specialized medical help. Most patients seek "the best expert," but they feel ill-equipped to evaluate doctors. They want to take charge of the decisions in cases where alternatives are available, but they are uncomfortable with the extent of their knowledge as a basis for making those decisions.

The combination of high expectations and defensive consumerism sets the stage for a new doctor-patient relationship. In seeking new forms of relating appropriate to the changing context of health care, doctor and patient will naturally strive for consistency with ethical principles already embedded deeply in the culture they share. They will debate in an arena that already honors the principle of telling the truth. But if there are to be exceptions to the rule of truth-telling, then the exceptions must be related to some consensus about the good of the individual or of society. Also, as we have seen, our culture generally respects the autonomy of the individual in making decisions about his or her own body and future. A discussion of the issues requires that we consider various circumstances: telling the whole truth; informed consent of individuals who are patients; and informed consent of individuals who are research subjects.

THE WHOLE TRUTH AND "THERAPEUTIC PRIVILEGE"

Both deontological and utilitarian moral philosophers have attempted to justify the principle of telling the truth. Immanuel Kant wrote an essay on the subject, titled "On the Supposed Right to Lie from Altruistic Motives," in which he argued that "the duty of being truthful . . . is uncondi-tional . . . to be truthful (honest) in all declarations, therefore is a sacred and absolutely commanding decree of reason, limited to no expediency."

For their part, utilitarians concentrate on the negative consequences of *not* telling the truth. They point to the destruction of trust, interaction, and cooperation. Utilitarians and deontologists alike stop short of absolute rules, claiming that telling the truth ought to be considered a prima facie duty—not a rule without legitimate exceptions.

From the perspective of a doctor who withholds information or tells a lie to a patient, the doctrine of "therapeutic privilege" or some similar moral reason concerning patient welfare allows the physician to set aside the normal duty of disclosure. Simply stated, this means that a doctor may permissibly convey less than the whole truth if he or she believes that an omission of information is in the patient's best therapeutic interests. The physician's primary responsibility, as viewed within the profession, is to the successful treatment of the patient. This rationale is accepted even though the patient effectively is excluded from decision-making because of the absence of accurate information.

"Therapeutic privilege" is the best-known legal provision allowing this form of physician nondisclosure. In the medical sphere, many physicians will hold that the principle "first, do no harm" (*primum non nocere*) frequently prevails over telling the truth. One important account of the strategy of maintaining therapeutic privilege was given in a 1957 court case:

The physician must place the welfare of his patient above all else and this very fact places him in a position in which he sometimes must choose between two alterna-tive courses of action. One is to explain to the patient every risk attendant upon any surgical procedure or operation, no matter how remote; this may well result in alarming a patient who is already unduly apprehensive and who as a result refuses to undertake surgery in which there is in fact minimum risk; it may also result in actually increasing the risks by reason of the physiological results of the apprehension itself. The other is to recognize that each patient presents a separate problem, that the patient's mental and emotional condition is important and in certain cases may be crucial, and that in discussing the element of risk a certain amount of discretion must be employed consistent with the full disclosure of facts necessary to informed consent.[1]

1. *Salgo* v. *Leland Stanford, Jr., University Bd. of Trustees*, 154 Cal. App. 2d 560, 317 P.2d 170 (1957).

Therapeutic privilege and physician nondisclosure in general are by no means universally accepted, though in the past they had more general acceptance than they do today. We will shortly see how it has recently become the exception rather than the rule that guides doctors when decisions are made about how much information to provide a patient. This shift, many believe, reflects a fundamental difference between the perspectives of health care professionals and of their patients regarding information about diagnoses and possible treatment.

For example, in a recent survey of physicians' disclosure practices in seizure management, physicians reported that they routinely disclose an average of five to six of a possible sixteen facts about the risks and side effects of seizure medication. By contrast, when seizure patients and parents of seizure patients were asked which facts they would want to be told, they reported wanting to be informed of an average of thirteen to fourteen facts.[2] These differences in perspective have resulted in a rapid increase in the number of lawsuits brought by patients against their doctors and hospitals. Some patients whose doctors have exercised a privilege to lie or withhold information now are suing their doctors for negligence (or, in rare cases, battery). In the past, patients who sued doctors and hospitals might have alleged "battery" by claiming a procedure was intentionally performed without their knowledge and permission. Today patients who bring a malpractice action tend to allege "negligence" by claiming they were not given adequate information. Both patients and medical professionals are becoming more cautious about entering into close relationships that in the past might have been approached with informal mutual trust and openness. To some extent, this may be symptomatic of a broader cultural development in which people have come to challenge authority and to suspect the motives of many, if not all, professionals. Certainly the grounds for objecting to deception and withholding of information are not narrowly legal; in their origin they are wholly moral grounds.

PATIENTS' RIGHTS

The right to self-determination has a long-standing tradition in Anglo-American law. This regard for individual persons includes his or her right to make free choices. Respect for self-determination underlies the American Declaration of Independence and its claim that all citizens are entitled to "Life, Liberty, and the Pursuit of Happiness." Self-determination in health care has a traditional basis in case law, as the following famous statement by Justice Cardozo in 1914 indicates:

2. Ruth Faden, et al., "Disclosure of Information to Patients in Medical Care," *Medical Care* 19 (July 1981): 718–33.

Every human being of adult years and sound mind has a right to determine what should be done with his own body; and a surgeon who performs an operation without his patient's consent commits an assault, for which he is liable in damages . . . this is true except in cases of emergency where the patient is unconscious and where it is necessary to operate before consent can be obtained.[3]

In 1960 two important cases led the way in malpractice suits alleging that the patient did not receive adequate information. Their combined result was to establish a common-law duty for the doctor to disclose to the patient all material risks involved in medical treatment. One case occurred in Missouri, where a patient brought an action for negligence due to bone fractures he received during convulsions as a side-effect of insulin shock treatments. The court decided:

In the particular circumstances of this record, considering the nature of Mitchell's illness and this rather new and radical procedure with its rather high incidence of serious and permanent injuries not connected with the illness, the doctors owed their patient in possession of his faculties the duty to inform him generally of the possible serious collateral hazards; and in the detailed circumstances there was a submissible fact issue of whether the doctors were negligent in failing to inform him of the dangers of shock therapy.[4]

The other important case in 1960 occurred in Kansas, where a patient brought a malpractice action against a physician and a hospital for injuries sustained as a result of cobalt radiation therapy after a radical mastectomy. In addition to alleging negligence of procedures, the plaintiff also charged that the physician failed to warn her of possible side effects during treatment. The court restated the concept of patient self-determination as articulated by Justice Cardozo in 1914 and decided that the physician was obligated to make a reasonable disclosure of known dangers in the proposed treatment:

Anglo-American law starts with the premise of thoroughgoing self-determination. It follows that each man is considered to be the master of his own body, and he may, if he be of sound mind, expressly prohibit the performance of life-saving surgery, or other medical treatment.[5]

These two cases had two important results, one legal, the other social. Legally, the concept of patient self-determination received sharp and significant restatement; and the obligations of physicians to inform patients of the results of treatment, including possible side effects, was explicitly established in the law. The social effect was to add to the dramatically

3. *Schloendorff* v. *Society of New York Hospital*, 105 N.E. 92 (N.Y., 1914).
4. *Mitchell* v. *Robinson*, 334 S.W. 2d 11 (Mo., 1960).
5. *Natanson* v. *Kline*, 187 Kan. 186, 354 P.2d 670 (1960).

increasing number of malpractice actions. According to James Ludlam, the frequency of informed consent cases went up, starting in the mid-1950s, "absolutely and relatively to nearly every other issue litigated in malpractice actions." He also quotes a major 1974 study as reporting that fourteen percent of malpractice cases brought alleged lack of informed consent. "However," he concludes, "it is believed that the practice of pleading the lack of informed consent has materially increased since the 1974 study."[6]

UNDER THE LAW, WHAT IS ADEQUATE DISCLOSURE?

In recent years the courts repeatedly have upheld the right of informed patients to refuse treatment and have continued to expand the notion of "the right to self-determination." In a court case in the 1970s, informed consent was explicated in terms of the responsibility of the health care professional "to explain the procedure to the patient and to warn him of any material risks or dangers inherent in or collateral to the therapy, so as to enable the patient to make an intelligent and informed choice about whether or not to undergo such treatment."[7]

The case of John Marx, with which we began this chapter, is one among thousands, and yet it fits a pattern of problems, based on an abuse of informed consent. Traditionally, courts have tended to protect physicians. They have supported the assumption that a physician, with superior knowledge, should decide how much information to give the patient. In cases in which a patient has sued a physician for withholding information, the court usually has instructed the jury to consider the opinions of other physicians in the community regarding adequacy of the disclosure. Expert medical testimony of this kind has either confirmed or denied that the information given to a patient was in conformity with "standard medical practice" in similar cases. In all but the truly extraordinary cases, expert medical witnesses have been reluctant to condemn the judgments and behavior of their colleagues. Thus, it has proved difficult to establish that a doctor had violated what was termed "prevailing standard practice."

In the ruling written in the case of *Natanson* v. *Kline* cited above, the court confirmed the customary limit of informed consent: "The duty of the physician to disclose, however, is limited to those disclosures which a reasonable medical practitioner would make under the same or similar circumstances." The professional practice standard thus entails that an

6. James Ludlam, *Informed Consent* (Chicago: American Hospital Association, 1978), p. 6.
7. *Sard* v. *Hardy*, 379 A.2d 1014, 1020 (Md., 1977).

adequate disclosure is one that reflects what a reasonable medical practitioner would disclose.

More recently, an increasing number of state, federal, and appellate courts (still not a majority) have shifted away from the criterion of "prevailing standard practice." According to the newer "reasonable person standard," the information necessary for informed consent is that which a "reasonable person" would expect to know about potential benefits, side effects, and risks of treatment. Three precedent-setting cases occurred in 1972: *Canterbury v. Spence*, 464 F.2d 772 (D.C. cir. 1972); *Cobbs v. Grant*, 8 Cal.3d 229, 502 P.2d 1, 104 Cal. Rpts. 505 (1972); and *Wilkinson v. Vesey*, 110 R.I. 606, 295 A.2d 676 (1972). In these cases, the courts rejected "prevailing practice" as the standard for informed consent, and ruled instead that the physician must disclose risks that are "material" to the patient's decision. A "material risk" is defined in *Canterbury* as one that "a reasonable person, in what the physician knows or should know to be the patient's position, would be likely to attach significance to in deciding whether or not to forego the proposed therapy." In reflecting on this definition, you may wish to think about John Marx again: Do you think that he would have had a better chance of winning his malpractice suit under one of these standards than the other?

The following chart will summarize the standards for determining when informed consent has been achieved or not achieved:

Competing Standards for Determining Informed Consent

- **STANDARD MEDICAL PRACTICE**
  A doctor is not wrong in withholding information if other doctors in the same area generally think he or she is doing the right thing. This is the longer standing and more generally accepted standard.

- **REASONABLE PERSON STANDARD**
  The "reasonable person" does not have to be a doctor or other health care professional. The shift is to the side of the patient. What would the reasonable person expect to know about his or her condition and choices in treatment? Emphasis is given to "material risks" that may attend various courses of action. This is the newer, less accepted, but growing standard.

The Primary Exceptions

- **THERAPEUTIC PRIVILEGE**
  The doctor knows best, and may withhold information if he or she thinks the information would run the risk of harming the patient.

- **EMERGENCY SITUATIONS**

A doctor need not obtain informed consent to provide emergency treatment to prevent loss of life or limb.

The shift now taking place in the standard for disclosure in matters of informed consent is in some ways a subtle one. It may seem more distinct and significant when you consider that it is a shift from an emphasis on a health care professional's *duty to disclose* information that he or she deems important to an emphasis on the patient's *rights of access* to information and to decision-making. It is easily possible to overdo this contrast, but the main point is that society is in the middle of an important shift in emphasis from physicians' judgments of their obligations to patients toward the rights that patients have to make informed choices.

Proponents of the "reasonable person standard" believe that it favors the patient's right of self-determination and that it recognizes the fact that a physician's medical expertise may be only one of several factors that are of value to the patient. Other things may be more important to an individual than his or her own physical well-being. Furthermore, proponents argue that "prevailing standard practice" may be difficult to determine with any accuracy and that some situations may be so new or unusual that physicians may have no common standard to which they can refer.

By contrast, those who favor the criterion of "prevailing standard practice" argue that medicine has become so complicated that *only* a doctor has the knowledge and perspective to weigh all the variables in planning treatment for a patient. Furthermore, they say, a "reasonable person standard" does not take into account the unique needs of each patient and can be dangerous to the patient's health.

OBTAINING INFORMED CONSENT

Because of the increased number of malpractice suits based on alleged lack of informed consent, health care professionals, their professional organizations, and hospitals have had to examine the means they use to make disclosure and to gain consent. In many health care settings it is regarded as sufficient for a patient to sign a general consent agreement upon entering a hospital. Now we commonly see new forms of disclosure, such as the use of videotapes, pamphlets, and patient interviews. Some hospitals provide brochures or even multimedia presentations as a means of conveying information to patients. We also see informed consent forms that apply to specific procedures. Often the forms include elaborate explanations or packets of information that the patient is supposed to read before signing the form. Physicians and nurses are cautioned to keep detailed records of what information they give to their patients, and when they give it.

These more elaborate consent procedures have been criticized by medical professionals, sociologists, educators, and language experts. For example, one study[8] surveyed 200 patients the day after they signed consent forms for chemotherapy, radiation therapy, or surgery. Sixty percent understood the purpose and nature of their signing the consent forms—a statistic some take to be good and others take to be ominous. Most patients thought the consent forms were meant to "protect the physician's rights"—a view that may, of course, be correct! T. M. Grundner analyzed five representative surgical consent forms by means of two standardized tests of readability[9] and found that four of the five forms were written "at the level of a scientific journal, and the fifth at the level of a specialized academic magazine." The problem of the readability of these forms (though not necessarily of the disclosures that precede their use) has for years been a notorious one in modern medicine.

Those who defend more specific and readable consent forms often cite a 1971 study by Ralph Alfidi. He studied consent forms used before angiography at the Cleveland Clinic Foundation. (Angiography is a diagnostic procedure to examine blood vessels made visible by injection of a substance that shows up on X ray. It is a procedure frequently accompanied by discomfort.) Alfidi discovered that the majority of the 232 patients desired and valued the information given to them in the consent forms. Of the 232 patients, 228 signed the form authorizing angiography. Alfidi said, "We believe that we have proven that the majority of patients not only have a right to know, but want to know what possible complications may be expected from any given procedure."[10]

'DOCTOR' SGANARELLE: Now these vapors I refer to, making a passage from the left side, where the liver is, to the right side, where the heart is, it comes about that the lungs, which we call in Latin *armyan*, having a communication with the brain, which we term in Greek *nasmus*, by means of the vena cava, which we denominate in Hebrew *cubile*, encounter on their path the aforesaid vapors, which fill the ventricles of the scapula; and because the aforesaid vapors have a certain malignity, which is caused by the acridity of the humors engendered in the concavity of the diaphragm, it then happens

8. Barrie Cassileth, Robert Zupkis, Katherine Sutton-Smith, and Vicki March, "Informed Consent—Why Are Its Goals Imperfectly Realized?" *New England Journal of Medicine* 302 (1980): 896–900.

9. T. M. Grundner, "On the Readability of Surgical Consent Forms," *New England Journal of Medicine* 302 (1980): 900–02.

10. Ralph Alfidi, "Informed Consent: A Study of Patient Reaction," *Journal of the American Medical Association* 216 (1971): 1325–29.

that the vapors—ossabundus, nequeys, nequer, potarinum, quipsa milus. And that is exactly how it comes about that your daughter is mute.

GERONE: I ask your pardon for my ignorance.

SGANARELLE: No harm done. You aren't obliged to be as well informed as we are.

—Molière,
The Physician in Spite of Himself

THE EMERGENCY SITUATION

In reflecting on the above discussion of the ethics of information transmitted from doctor to patient, you probably have been thinking in terms of the conventional doctor-patient encounter. A patient seeks counsel from a doctor in order to deal with troublesome symptoms, or else to get a routine checkup. After diagnostic procedures the doctor becomes aware of something which he or she may or may not share with the patient. By now, you are devloping your own views about doctors' prerogatives and patients' rights in these matters, and it is time for us to turn attention to less conventional circumstances. Take, for example, the situations that arise in emergency rooms. In practice, a special set of rules applies there, despite the growing number of patients who have no family doctor and are seeking routine treatment in emergency rooms. Because emergency situations frequently involve unconscious patients or those in trauma, who are incapable of informed decision-making, doctors and nurses must stand ready to make decisions for the patients without consulting anyone. In such emergencies, the courts have not insisted on informed consent from the patient or the family, although it has recommended family consultation.

In the case of *Canterbury* v. *Spence,* the court provided a definition of "emergency": ". . . the patient is unconscious or otherwise incapable of consenting, and harm from a failure to treat is imminent and outweighs any harm threatened by the proposed treatment." Some writers have argued that the professional ought to treat an "emergency patient" by the criterion of a "reasonable person." The concept is a simple application of the reasonable person standard discussed earlier; it says that doctors should do that which the average reasonable person would be likely to want done in a particular emergency.

CONSENT TO MEDICAL RESEARCH ON HUMANS

Another special set of circumstances surrounds the person recruited for medical research. In the basic investigation of an illness and possibly effective new treatments for that illness, it becomes necessary at some point to test procedures of these emerging new theories and techniques. Medical researchers need the cooperation of individuals who will be exposed to medical risks for the sake of science and ultimately for the sake of future patients who will be the beneficiaries of scientific discoveries.

The problem is that potential subjects of research may be in poor condition to resist the invitation to participate. Prisoners and the desperately ill are cases in point. In order to protect these people from undue pressure or misleading information from experimenters, the government has in recent years set forth strict guidelines and procedures for gaining informed consent from these patients and research subjects. One fear is that many researchers are so eager to prove their theories, and thereby potentially provide benefit to many people, that they will "blur the facts" when explaining experiments and risks to potential subjects.

In the past, researchers' dedication to science has sometimes prompted them to experiment on people entirely without their knowledge or permission. As soon as these experiments started to reach public awareness, a debate ensued that continues to this day. The public and its official leadership demanded new policies regarding informed consent for medical research. This heightened concern for a more formal and consistent relationship between medical researchers and their human subjects, of course, directly parallels the previously noted concerns about the relationship between doctor and patient.

No example has done more to sensitize us about the need for consent and the possibility of abuse than the disclosures at the Nuremberg trials after World War II. In the course of these trials of certain Nazi leaders some grisly stories came to public attention. Here was abuse in the extreme. Nazi medical researchers performed sometimes bizarre medical experiments on concentration camp victims without their consent, and indeed absolutely against their will. The physical and emotional damage inflicted upon human subjects was of little concern to the researchers, and the purpose of an "investigation" often was either unclear or tended to duplicate prior findings. One result of the public awareness of the Nuremberg trials was the adoption of the Nuremberg Code, whose first rule bears on informed consent:

The voluntary consent of the human subject is absolutely essential. This means that the person involved should have legal capacity to give consent; should be so situated as to be able to exercise free power of choice, without the intervention of any element of force, fraud, deceit, duress, overreaching, or other ulterior form of constraint or coercion; and should have sufficient knowledge and comprehension of the elements of the subject matter involved as to enable him to make an understanding and enlightened decision. This latter element requires that before the acceptance of an affirmative decision by the experimental subject, there should be made known to him the nature, duration, and purpose of the experiment; the method and means by which it is to be conducted; all inconveniences and hazards reasonably to be expected; and the effects upon his health or person which may possibly come from his participation in the experiment.[11]

In 1964, the World Medical Assembly adopted the Declaration of Helsinki, which confirmed the essence of the first rule of the Nuremberg Code and made even more detailed stipulations about consent.

The problems of consent explored in the Nuremberg trials were not merely the outcome of certain Nazi excesses. Problems of consent to experimentation have long plagued even the highest echelons of American medicine. For example, in 1963 it was reported that senile elderly patients had been injected with live cancer cells for a study at the Jewish Chronic Disease Hospital in Brooklyn, New York, in collaboration with researchers from the prestigious Sloan-Kettering Institute. There was a public outcry, a nasty trial, and a loss by some physicians of their licenses to practice medicine. In a second case in New York State, at the Willowbrook State Hospital School, a study of hepatitis included actively inoculating mentally retarded children with hepatitis virus.

The U.S. Public Health Service addressed some of these issues in 1966 and 1968, when it published guidelines requiring consent in federally supported drug research. By 1974, the guidelines became official regulations enforced by the then Department of Health, Education, and Welfare (now Department of Health and Human Services). Since then, all federally funded experimentation on humans required approval by a local review committee that was charged with evaluating the adequacy of the protections for human subjects found in every piece of research reviewed. Thus, since the early 1970s, major medical centers have had committees called Institutional Review Boards (IRBs). These boards oversee research proposals and preside over the methods for obtaining human subjects. The boards are charged with the responsibility to assure that subjects give adequately informed consent and that the scientific benefits of the research justify risks to individuals. These boards typically include among their memberships lawyers, ethicists, and other nonmedical representatives.

Ironically, it was reported in 1971 that during the 1930s Public Health Service doctors themselves deliberately had withheld treatment from a group of rural black men suffering from syphilis in Tuskegee, Alabama. The research purpose was to observe the "natural history" of the untreated

11. *Trials of War Criminals before the Nuremberg Military Tribunals under Control Council Law No. 10*, vol. 2, (Nuremberg, October 1946–April 1949). Available in Tom L. Beauchamp and LeRoy Walters, eds., *Contemporary Issues in Bioethics* (Belmont, Calif.: Dickenson Publishing Co., 1978), pp. 404–05.

disease of syphilis. The Department of Health, Education, and Welfare sponsored an investigation of the incident, and a report was issued in 1973. The report influenced the search for public policy:

Human experimentation reflects the recurrent societal dilemma of reconciling respect for human rights and individual dignity with the felt needs of society to overrule individual autonomy for the common good. Throughout this report we have expressed our concern for the lack of attention which has been given to the protection of the rights and welfare of human subjects in research. Society can no longer afford to leave the balancing of individual rights against scientific progress to the scientific community alone. The revelations of the Tuskegee Syphilis Study once again dramatically confirmed this conclusion.

We offer our far-reaching proposals in the hope that the decision-making process for human research will become more open and more effectively regulated. We have amply documented the need for implementing this most basic recommendation. Precise rules and efficient procedures are not by themselves proof against a repetition of Tuskegee for, however well designed the system of regulation, the danger of token adherence to ethical standards and evasion in the guise of flexibility will persist. Ultimately the spirit in which an aware society undertakes to use human beings for research ends will determine the protection which these human beings will receive. Therefore we have urged throughout a greater participation by society in the decisions which affect so many human lives.[12]

In 1974 the U.S. Congress passed the National Research Act, which led directly to the establishment of the National Commission for the Protection of Human Subjects of Biomedical and Behavioral Research. The commission has had considerable influence. After studying the issues in some depth, it issued several reports and recommendations to Congress and to the Secretary of Health and Human Services. Within 180 days after receipt of its recommendations, Health and Human Services was required to adopt the recommendations or publish reasons for not doing so. The smattering of examples below, which paraphrase a few commission recommendations to Congress, demonstrate that our society is beginning to translate moral concern into public policy in this area.

Some of the commission's recommendations to the Secretary of the Department of Health and Human Services (then DHEW), *as they pertain to matters of informed consent,* are as follows:

Research on the fetus. On July 25, 1975 the commission forwarded recommendations to the secretary that later deeply influenced the formulation of government guidelines. Among its recommendations, the commission proposed that various forms of both therapeutic and non-

12. Department of Health, Education and Welfare, *Final Report of the Tuskegee Syphilis Study Ad Hoc Advisory Panel,* April 28, 1973 (Washington, D.C.: U.S. Government Printing Office, 1973, #747–022/5334), p. 47.

therapeutic research on the fetus could be performed, but that when directed toward the pregnant woman, research could proceed only if the woman had given her informed consent. In some cases the commission held that the research should occur only if the father has not objected.[13]

Research on children. The commission forwarded its recommendations on September 6, 1977. The recommendations approved minimal-risk research involving children and also approved more-than-minimal-risk research under certain conditions, when it is "presented by an intervention that holds out the prospect of direct benefit for the individual subjects, or by a monitoring procedure required for the well being of the subjects." To insure proper protections, the commission recommended a variety of mechanisms for assuring that the permission of parents and the assent of children (when applicable) is free and informed. The commission took the general view that the assent of children should be solicited when they are capable of assenting and that a parent, guardian, or similar protective source should also give an informed consent.[14] (The commission also held that the objection of children to nontherapeutic research could under some conditions be decisive.)

Research on prisoners. The commission forwarded its recommendations on October 1, 1976. It recommended that prisoners should not be the subjects of nontherapeutic research (generally drug research) unless "compelling" reasons for using prisoners were involved, conditions of "equity" were satisfied, and there was a significant degree of free consent by the prisoners. Since the commission did not believe that such free consent was generally possible in the coercive atmosphere of prisons as we now know them, it recommended that prison research be discontinued until such conditions could be present.[15]

Research on the institutionalized mentally infirm. These recommendations were forwarded on February 2, 1978. The commission recommended in effect that this class of subjects be provided similar protections to those it had earlier suggested for children, but it went on to suggest even more stringent protections. It was thought that some subjects are capable of consenting, whereas others are not. If the subject could not consent (or even assent or dissent) in the case of nontherapeutic research, and a

13. National Commission for the Protection of Human Subjects of Biomedical and Behavioral Research, *Report and Recommendations: Research on the Fetus* (Washington, D.C.: U.S. Department of Health, Education, and Welfare, 1975), pp. 73–76.

14. National Commission for the Protection of Human Subjects of Biomedical and Behavioral Research, *Report and Recommendations: Research Involving Children* (Washington, D.C.: U.S. Department of Health, Education, and Welfare, 1977), pp. 1–20.

15. National Commission for the Protection of Human Subjects of Biomedical and Behavioral Research, *Report and Recommendations: Research Involving Prisoners* (Washington, D.C.: U.S. Department of Health, Education, and Welfare, 1976), pp. 14–21.

certain level of risk were attained, the commission recommended that a guardian of the person must give permission. (Other, more complicated consent recommendations were filed in the case of a mentally infirm person who objected to *therapeutic* research.)[16]

In the case of prisoners in particular, authorities have been concerned that prisoners might be unduly influenced in submitting to medical experimentation in hopes of gaining special favor, or simply to relieve boredom. Also, it is reasonable to wonder whether some prisoners carry sufficiently high self-esteem to protect themselves from physical danger. Recently, experimentation among prisoners has been curtailed sharply. The National Commission's report, as noted, argued that the captive status of prisoners reduced their capacity for autonomy and opened the way for abuses of authoritarianism by prison officials and inducements offered by drug company representatives. This set of conclusions has been debated, however, and federal officials recently have been involved in a perpetual process of reconsidering the issues.

We have not yet achieved clear guidelines to deal with the problem of consent among children, adolescents, the very old, and many other "vulnerable" populations. In each case the problem is to define the extent to which the individual can understand the research proposition described to him or her and make an intelligent decision. Doubts about very young children can hardly be controversial, but it is more difficult to decide when an adult of advanced years is able to make a decision autonomously. Our society faces a fascinating challenge in balancing the great need for human experimental subjects against the ethical requirements to protect human subjects from unfair exploitation, danger, and loss of self-determination.

A NATIONAL FORUM

Serious concern for bioethical issues began largely after World War II. Today the debate continues in courts, government agencies, universities, and the general public. As we write this volume, thoughtful people are discovering the wide range of issues that deserve consideration. Almost all general-circulation magazines and newspapers frequently report cases involving bioethical issues, and these subjects have become the staple of novels, television and motion picture dramas, electronic journalism, and international conferences. Even if you had not noticed it before, reading

16. National Commission for the Protection of Human Subjects of Biomedical and Behavioral Research, *Report and Recommendations: Research Involving Those Institutionalized as Mentally Infirm* (Washington, D.C.: U.S. Department of Health, Education, and Welfare, 1978), pp. 1–22.

this book will lead you to notice that, in its media and public forums, our society is wrestling with bioethical issues as never before.

Largely as a result of the arousal of public concern, and in part also because of the work of the National Commission for the Protection of Human Subjects, in 1979 President Carter established a new President's Commission for the Study of Ethical Problems in Medicine and Biomedical and Behavioral Research. This new commission in effect replaced both the old National Commission (which was active from 1974 to 1978) and the old Department of Health, Education, and Welfare's Ethics Advisory Board (which was active from 1977 to 1980). The commission continued in the Reagan Administration to deal with many of the questions discussed in this book. Its activities, in a sense, served as the focal point of a national public debate in the United States.

COPING WITH AND SHAPING CHANGES

Achieving informed consent, we have now seen, includes these elements:

1. exchange of information from health care practitioner to patient;
2. deliberation about what is adequate information and about how much information may be detrimental;
3. debate about the best means to obtain true informed consent;
4. increased activity by individual patients and special interest groups in the society to seek informed consent;
5. a slight but noteworthy shift in the courts as to what makes up informed consent from peer evaluation among physicians to an estimate of what any reasonable person in a similar situation would want to know;
6. greatly increased activity of the federal government to protect certain populations;
7. establishment of IRBs, which include medical scientists and nonscientists in key decision-making roles.

These developments and the new "Principles of Medical Ethics" issued by the AMA in 1981, which for the first time admonishes the physician to "respect the rights of patients," are among the visible signs of a major values transition in our society.

It is neither accurate nor especially helpful to designate simplistic categories of people in the current debate. Health care practitioners, patients, citizens, professional organizations, and special interest groups are grappling with these complex issues. We all sense that the ground is shifting under accepted norms and practices. Perhaps a way to describe this shift of values is as the beginning of a more sophisticated and enlightened use of the prerogatives of health care professionals and, at the same time, clearer and more assertive use of self-determination by patients and the general citizenry.

SELECTED READINGS
Informed Consent—A "Canon of Loyalty"? . . .[17]

One need not read very far in medical ethics—and especially not in the literature concerning medical experimentation or the ethical "codes" that have been formulated since the medical cases at the Nuremberg trials—without realizing that medical ethics has not its sole basis in the overall benefits to be produced. It is not a consequence-ethics alone. It is not solely a teleological ethics, to use the language of philosophy. It is not even an ethics of the "greatest possible medical benefits for the greatest possible number" of people. That calculus too easily comes to mean the "greatest possible medical benefits regardless of the number" of patients who without their proper consent may be made the subjects of promising medical investigations. Medical ethics is not solely a benefit-producing ethics even in regard to the individual patient, since he should not always be helped without his will.

As stated in the *Ethical Guidelines for Organ Transplantation* of the American Medical Association, so also of medical experimentation involving human subjects: "Man participates in these procedures: he is the patient in them; or he performs them. All mankind is the ultimate beneficiary of them." Observe that the respect in which man is the patient and man the performer of medical care or medical investigation (the relation between doctor and patient/subject) places an independent moral limit upon the fashion in which the rest of mankind can be made the ultimate beneficiary of these procedures. In the language of philosophy, a deontological dimension or test holds chief place in medical ethics, beside teleological considerations. That is to say, there must be a determination of the rightness or wrongness of the action and not only of the good to be obtained in medical care or from medical investigation.

A crucial element in answer to the question, What constitutes right action in medical practice? is the requirement of a reasonably free and adequately informed consent. In current medical ethics, this is a chief *canon of loyalty* (as I shall call it) between the man who is patient/subject and the man who performs medical investigational procedures. Physicians discuss the consent-requirement just as ethicists discuss fairness—or justice-claims: these tests must be satisfied along with the benefits (the "good") obtained. . . .

Hopefully while not exceeding an ethicist's putative competence or trespassing upon the competence of medical men, I wish to undertake an analysis of the consent-requirement itself. The principle of an informed consent is a statement of the fidelity between the man who performs medical procedures and the man on whom they are performed. Other aspects of medical ethics—for example, the

17. Excerpts from Paul Ramsey, *The Patient as Person* (New Haven: Yale University Press, 1970), pp. 2, 5, 8–11.

requirement of a good experimental design and of professional skill at least as good as is customary in ordinary medical practice—treat the man as a purely passive subject or patient. These are also the requirements that hold for an ethical experiment upon animals. But any human being is more than a patient or experimental subject; he is a personal subject—every bit as much a man as the physician-investigator. Fidelity is between man and man in these procedures. Consent expresses or establishes this relationship, and the requirement of consent sustains it. Fidelity is the bond between consenting man and consenting man in these procedures. The principle of an informed consent is the cardinal *canon of loyalty* joining men together in medical practice and investigation. In this requirement, faithfulness among men—the faithfulness that is normative for all the covenants or moral bonds of life with life—gains specification for the primary relations peculiar to medical practice.

Consent as a canon of loyalty can best be exhibited by a paraphrase of Reinhold Niebuhr's celebrated defense of democracy on both positive and negative grounds: "Man's capacity for justice makes democracy possible; man's propensity to injustice makes democracy necessary."[a] Man's capacity to become joint adventurers in a common cause makes the consensual relation possible; man's propensity to overreach his joint adventurer even in a good cause makes consent necessary. In medical experimentation the common cause of the consensual relation is the advancement of medicine and benefit to others. In therapy and in diagnostic or therapeutic investigations, the common cause is some benefit to the patient himself; but this is still a joint venture in which patient and physician can say and ideally should both say, "I cure."

Therefore, I suggest that men's capacity to become joint adventurers in a common cause makes possible a consent to enter the relation of patient to physician or of subject to investigator. This means that *partnership* is a better term than *contract* in conceptualizing the relation between patient and physician or between subject and investigator. The fact that these pairs of people are joint adventurers is evident from the fact that consent is a continuing and a repeatable requirement. We can legitimately appeal to permissions presumably granted by or implied in the original contract only to the extent that these are not incompatible with the demands of an ongoing partnership sustained by an actual or implied present consent and terminable by any present or future dissent from it. For this to be at all a human enterprise—a covenantal relation between the man who performs these procedures and the man who is patient in them—the latter must make a reasonably free and an adequately informed consent. Ideally, he must be constantly engaged in doing so. This is basic to the cooperative enterprise in which he is one partner. . . .

The foregoing paragraphs describe the basis of the requirement that experimentation involving human subjects should be undertaken only when an informed consent has been secured. There are enormous problems, of course, in knowing how to subsume cases under this moral regulation expressive of respect

a. Reinhold Niebuhr, *The Children of Light and the Children of Darkness* (New York: Scribner's, 1949), p. xi.

for the man who is the subject in medical investigations no less than in applying this same moral regulation expressive of the meaning of medical care. What is and what is not a mature and informed consent is a preciously subtle thing to determine. Then there are questions about how to apply this rule arising from those sorts of medical research in which the patient's knowing enough to give an informed consent may alter the findings sought; and there is debate about whether the use of prisoners or medical students in medical experimentation, or paying the participants, would not put them under too much duress for them to be said to consent freely even if fully informed. Despite these ambiguities, however, to obtain an understanding consent is a minimum obligation of a common enterprise and in practice in which men are committed to men in definable respects. The *faithfulness*-claims which every man, simply by being a man, places upon the researcher are the morally relevant considerations. This is the ground of the consent-rule in medical practice, though obviously medical practice has also its consequence-features.

. . . Or an "Elaborate Ritual"?[18]

. . . [T]he chances are remote that the subject really understands what he has consented to—in the sense that the responsible medical investigator understands the goals, nature, and hazards of his study. . . . It is moreover quite unlikely that any patient-subject can see himself accurately within the broad context of the situation, to weigh the inconveniences and hazards that he will have to undergo against the improvements that the research project may bring to the management of his disease in general and to his own case in particular. . . .

Nor can the information given to the experimental subject be in any sense totally complete. It would be impractical and probably unethical for the investigator to present the nearly endless list of all possible contingencies; in fact, he may not himself be aware of every untoward thing that might happen. . . .

Ideally, the subject should give his consent freely, under no duress whatsoever. The facts are that some element of coercion is instrumental in any investigator-subject transaction. Volunteers for experiments will usually be influenced by hopes of obtaining better grades, earlier parole, more substantial egos, or just mundane cash. These pressures, however, are but fractional shadows of those enclosing the patient-subject. . . . When "informed consent" is obtained, it is not the student, the destitute bum, or the prisoner to whom, by virtue of his condition, the thumb screws of coercion are most relentlessly applied; it is the most used and useful of all experimental subjects, the patient with disease.

When a man or woman agrees to act as an experimental subject, therefore, his or her consent is marked by neither adequate understanding nor total freedom of choice. The conditions of the agreement are a far cry from those visualized as ideal. Jonas would have the subject identify with the investigative endeavor so that he and the researcher would be seeking a common cause; "Ultimately, the appeal for volunteers should seek . . . free and generous endorsement, the appropriation

18. Excerpts from Franz Ingelfinger, editorial, "Informed (But Uneducated) Consent," excerpted by permission of the *New England Journal of Medicine* 287 (1972): 465–66.

of the research purpose into the person's [i.e., the subject's] own scheme of ends."[a] For Ramsey, "informed consent" should represent a "covenantal bond between consenting man and consenting man that makes them . . . joint adventurers in medical care and progress."[b] Clearly, to achieve motivations and attitudes of this lofty type, an educated and understanding, rather than merely informed, consent is necessary. . . .

The procedure currently approved in the United States for enlisting human experimental subjects has one great virtue: patient-subjects are put on notice that their management is in part at least an experiment. The deceptions of the past are no longer tolerated. Beyond this accomplishment, however, the process of obtaining "informed consent," with all its regulations and conditions, is no more than elaborate ritual, a device that, when the subject is uneducated and uncomprehending, confers no more than the semblance of propriety on human experimentation. The subject's only real protection, the public as well as the medical profession must recognize, depends on the conscience and compassion of the investigator and his peers.

The Harmful Effects of Being Informed[19]

Before human subjects are enrolled in experimental studies, a variety of preliminary rituals are now required. These include an explanation of the nature of the experimental procedure and a specific elaboration of possible adverse reactions. The subjects, in turn, can either withdraw from the experiment or give their "informed consent." These rituals are said to increase the subjects' understanding of the procedures but, perhaps more important, they came into existence because of a strong belief in the fundamental principle that human beings have the right to determine what will be done to their minds and bodies.

Some, on the other hand, consider that the purpose of informed consent is not protection of subjects, but rather protection of investigators and sponsoring institutions from lawsuits based on the charge of subject deception should a misadventure result. But lawsuits arise in any case; subjects simply claim that they did not understand the rituals. It is reasonable, then, to ask whether the putative beneficiary, the subject, might be harmed rather than helped by the current informed consent procedure.

A considerable body of psychological evidence indicates that humans are highly suggestible. Information has been found to change people's attitudes, to change their moods and feelings, and even to make them believe they have experienced events that never in fact occurred. This alone would lead one to suspect that adverse reactions might result from information given during an informed consent discussion.

a. H. Jonas, "Philosophical Reflections on Experimenting with Human Subjects," *Daedalus* 98 (Spring 1969): 219–47.

b. Paul Ramsey, "The Ethics of a Cottage Industry in an Age of Community and Research Medicine," *New England Journal of Medicine* 284 (1971): 700–06.

19. Excerpts from Elizabeth Loftus and James F. Fries, "Informed Consent May Be Hazardous to Health," *Science* 204 (1979), p. 11 (copyright 1979 by the American Association for the Advancement of Science).

An examination of the medical evidence demonstrates that there is also a dark side to the placebo effect. Not only can positive therapeutic effects be achieved by suggestion, but negative side effects and complications can similarly result. For example, among subjects who participated in a drug study after the usual informed consent procedure, many of those given an injection of a placebo reported physiologically unlikely symptoms such as dizziness, nausea, vomiting, and even mental depression. One subject given the placebo reported that these effects were so strong that they caused an automobile accident. Many other studies provide similar data indicating that to a variable but often scarifying degree, explicit suggestion of possible adverse effects causes subjects to experience these effects. Recent hypotheses that heart attack may follow coronary spasm indicate physiological mechanisms by which explicit suggestions, and the stress that may be produced by them, might prove fatal. Thus, the possible consequences of suggested symptoms range from minor annoyance to, in extreme cases, death.

If protection of the subject is the reason for obtaining informed consent, the possibility of iatrogenic harm [harm actually caused by therapeutic treatment by a physician] to the subject as a direct result of the consent ritual must be considered. This clear cost must be weighed against the potential benefit of giving some people an increased sense of freedom of choice about the use of their bodies. The current legalistic devices, which are designed in part to limit subject recourse, intensify rather than solve a dilemma.

The features of informed consent procedures that do protect subjects should be retained. Experimental procedures should be reviewed by peers and public representatives. A statement to the subject describing the procedure and the general level of risk is reasonable. But detailed information should be reserved for those who request it. Specific slight risks, particularly those resulting from common procedures, should not be routinely disclosed to all subjects. And when a specific risk is disclosed, it should be discussed in the context of placebo effects in general, why they occur, and how to guard against them. A growing literature indicates that just as knowledge of possible symptoms can cause those symptoms, so can knowledge of placebo effects be used to defend against those effects. A move in this direction may ensure that a subject will not be at greater risk from self-appointed guardians than from the experiment itself.

ANNOTATED BIBLIOGRAPHY
Books and Articles

Barber, Bernard. *Informed Consent in Medical Therapy and Research*. New Brunswick, N.J.: Rutgers University Press, 1980. A medical sociologist looks at issues of informed consent, with an emphasis on the context of consent and of patient-physician or subject-investigator interaction.

Beauchamp, Tom L., and James F. Childress. *Principles of Biomedical Ethics*. New York: Oxford University Press, 1979. Chap. 3. This chapter gives philosophical background to the issue of informed consent by relating it to a moral "principle" of autonomy. The chapter also discusses informed refusal and autonomous suicide.

Canada Law Reform Commission. *Consent to Medical Care.* A monograph prepared by Margaret A. Somerville. Ottawa: Canadian Government Publication, 1979. This legal perspective also includes moral arguments. It focuses on developments in both Canadian and United States law.

Miller, Leslie J. "Informed Consent." *Journal of the American Medical Association* 244 (1980): 2100–03, 2347–50, 2556–58, 2661–62. This series of four integrated articles conveniently outlines recent developments in the literature of informed consent—with the positions of physicians in the law foremost in mind.

Veatch, Robert M. *A Theory of Medical Ethics.* New York: Basic Books, 1981. A sweeping book that stresses patient autonomy and rights in the context of medical practice.

Anthologies

Beauchamp, Tom L., and LeRoy Walters, eds. *Contemporary Issues in Bioethics.* 2nd ed. Belmont, Calif.: Wadsworth Publishing Company, 1982. Chaps. 4, 5, and 11. A standard anthology with lengthy introductions and carefully selected and edited articles. These three chapters focus respectively on patients' rights and professional obligations, disclosures in medical practice, and research with human subjects.

Robison, Wade L., and Michael S. Pritchard, eds. *Medical Responsibility: Paternalism, Informed Consent, and Euthanasia.* Clifton, N.J.: Humana Press, 1979. A good but heterogeneous collection of essays, with an emphasis on problems in the paternalistic treatment of patients.

Articles from the *Encyclopedia of Bioethics*

Informed Consent in Human Research
 I. Social Aspects *Bradford H. Gray*
II. Ethical and Legal Aspects *Karen Lebacqz and Robert J. Levine*
Informed Consent in Mental Health *Robert A. Burt*
Informed Consent in the Therapeutic Relationship
 I. Clinical Aspects *Eric J. Cassell*
II. Legal and Ethical Aspects *Jay Katz*
Rights
 I. Systematic Analysis *Joel Feinberg*
II. Rights in Bioethics *Ruth Macklin*
Truth-Telling
 I. Attitudes *Robert M. Veatch*
II. Ethical Aspects *Sissela Bok*

Literature

Williams, William Carlos. "The Use of Force." 1938. In *The Farmer's Daughters.* New York: New Directions, 1961. Probably America's best physician-writer, Williams's short story about a doctor's treatment of and relationship with a three-year-old girl reveals much about the elements of the doctor-patient relationship, including the reasons for forcing treatment on her: "The damned little brat must be protected against her own idiocy. . . . It is a social necessity."

Audio/Visual

"Are You Doing This for Me, Doctor, Or Am I Doing It for You?" "NOVA" series, 52-minute film or videotape. Sale or rental, Time/Life Video, Eisenhower Drive, Paramus, N.J., 07652. This episode questions whether true informed consent can be obtained when the doctor-patient relationship is so unequal and procedures may be performed for the sake of the doctor's new knowledge or experience rather than for the patient's well-being.

6

HEALTH AND THE "RIGHT" TO HEALTH

In preceding chapters we have seen that the *medical* choices made possible by developments in modern medicine have led to the necessity to make difficult *moral* choices. Usually, these are not clear-cut choices between good and evil, right and wrong, but rather are more difficult choices between two or more alternatives that have serious moral arguments in their support.

As we face such choices individually, we face them also collectively as a society. So profound are the implications of modern medical technology that they call out for the consensus generally achieved through accepted public policy. Such policy is made through the legislative and judicial actions of government. It is influenced by the political process of elections and through the lobbying activities of various groups. In forming its public policies, a society makes it choices. To the extent that it is possible to do so, it attempts to act out in these policies the general principles and attitudes that it values. Our society has held dear the principles of individual rights *and* the promotion of the "general welfare," for example. Translating these objectives into concrete laws and guidelines requires much deliberation. Officially as a society, we must decide to fund certain research and to leave other research unfunded. Once a medical technology has developed, we may decide to permit or prohibit its use in certain ways. Public policy can guide the activities of researchers and indirectly determine the boundaries of private decision-making for each individual in the society.

In this and remaining chapters, we focus on some of the important choices we face as a society. In matters of modern medicine, the issues and debates suggested here have deep and wide implications for us all—the outcomes of public policy debate frequently determine who may enjoy what level of health care, who may live, and who will die. Already we have made some "decisions," as demonstrated by the fact that, for example, low infant mortality rates, better health, and longer life are associated with people who are relatively wealthy, are white, and live in metropolitan areas.

Issues of personal access to modern medical developments and health care can be discussed in terms of humanitarian concern and democratic ideals, but such discussions cannot long ignore the fact that medical developments and medical treatments are *expensive*. For example, we have every reason to expect that one day there will be a fully functional artificial heart. By the time it is used routinely, tens of millions of dollars will have been spent in its research and development. Even beyond that initial cost, the heart itself, together with the surgical implantation and postoperative care required, would cost tens of thousands of dollars per individual receiving the new device. In almost all instances, these costs would be shared broadly among the population by ways of taxes or medical insurance premiums. Right now, we all provide tax money for government-sponsored research directed toward developing such an artificial heart. Escalating medical costs for research and care are taking a larger and larger slice of the economic pie in this society. Health care costs are rising at a rate faster than the rate of overall inflation is rising, and Social Security, Medicare, and Medicaid are jointly becoming among the largest items in the federal budget. At the same time, people are living longer, so there is an increasing demand for health care resources to assist the aged.

Not all health-related costs are direct. A number of programs are designed to reduce the incidence of serious illness. For example, we devote some of our national resources to expensive programs intended to diminish toxic pollutants in the environment, reduce cigarette smoking, improve nutrition, remove health hazards from work environments, and so on. The costs can be staggering. Clean air, for example, certainly can reduce the potential health threats for the general population. On the other hand, it is very expensive to develop, install, and monitor devices to achieve this end.

In recent years, our society has been involved in a tug-of-war between people who rank priorities differently. Pulling in one direction are those who want more studies, more regulations, and greater efforts to prevent health hazards to the general public. Pulling in the opposite direction are those who argue that constraints on manufacturers, for example, can hurt us all by reducing productive efficiency in factories while at the same time driving up costs. They point out that these costs must be passed along to the consumer in the form of higher prices. In this way the costs of eliminating or limiting environmental threats to health are paid by the consumer and a greater proportion of our total economic wealth goes to nonproductive activity, namely decreasing alleged threats to public health.

Others counter that decreasing threats to public health will eventually mean less money spent on treating the debilitating ill health that may result. This debate is only one example of the many considerations to be taken into account as our society decides how much of its total wealth to allocate for health care—indirectly, as when we allocate money to be spent on limiting environmental threats to well-being, or directly, as when we allocate funds for research or governmental health insurance programs such as Medicare. Decisions about what portion of our total economic pie goes to health are referred to as questions of *macroallocation*.

An editorial from the *Washington Post*, entitled "High Costs of Health," discusses some of the choices emerging in the public debate in which we are now involved:

With a Senate subcommittee deciding when human life begins, and a presidential commission recommending a uniform legal definition of when it ends, the trustees of the Medicare program reminded us last week that, tough as these issues may be, there are harder ones still to be addressed in keeping the organism healthy between these two signal events.

Medicare, the health insurance program covering most aged and disabled persons, is headed for hard times in the next decade and beyond. Already the program's costs have grown enormously—from about $7 billion in 1970 to over $40 billion this year. They will probably double again in the next five or six years. While much of this growth is tied to increases in general prices and wages, the trustees' report points to another factor of almost equal importance to the program—increases in the number and type of services provided to each patient. In other words, one major reason that medical costs have grown so rapidly—and are likely to keep growing even if the general price level stabilizes—is that people are getting more and fancier care.

The country now devotes almost 10 percent of its gross product to health care. That covers everything from corn pads to kidney dialysis, but hospital care is far and away the biggest and fastest growing item. People go to hospitals more, and spend more money while they're there, not because they like the accommodations but because, thanks to modern technology, there are many more types of diagnostic and treatment services that hospitals can provide, and these things are extremely expensive. While other things like diet, not smoking and modern sanitation are far more important contributors to general health than medical care, 10 percent of the GNP is probably not too much to be spending for the many benefits of modern medicine. As that percentage creeps up, however, as it is likely to do if present trends continue, the questions of how much is enough to spend on medical care and what to spend it on will come to be posed more sharply.

One school of thought holds that these difficult questions can be avoided by trying to make the medical market work better—limiting insurance coverage, for example, so that people pay more attention to prices in deciding whether to seek medical care and from what source. Recent pilot programs do show that requiring more cost-sharing by patients somewhat limits the use of medical care, at least among the non-aged. Whether that affects their health hasn't yet been determined. In any case, there are obvious limits to this approach. When you or your child is the one with the failing kidney, heart defect or rapidly spreading cancer, it's not likely that you'll be shopping around for the cheapest doctor or hospital rather than the very best one you can get.

Past administrations have tried in various ways—physician review groups, health planning agencies and direct cost controls—to get a hold on medical costs. The Reagan administration thus far proposes only to shift part of the cost burden to other levels of government or to individuals. Shifting the costs of caring for the very sick and the aged, with their generally limited resources, won't make them go away. A better solution is needed for what is rapidly becoming one of the country's major policy dilemmas.[1]

DEFINING HEALTH—OUR EXPECTATIONS

As the *cost* of health care has escalated, our *expectations* of medicine have expanded. It seems that the more successful medicine becomes, the more we expect from it. In some quarters, the definition of health has expanded to include an all-inclusive concern for human well-being—physical, mental, and social. At the same time, the demands of "rights" to health and health care have been extended to all segments of the population. Agencies of the United Nations and other organizations have claimed that this inclusive concept of health is a universal right "for all persons."

By the end of the 1970s, our growing expectations crashed into the realization that our resources were limited. Throughout the 1980s and into the foreseeable future, we must face difficult choices. Ostensibly, these choices are economic and political ones to be made through the legislative procedures of an open, democratic society. However, underlying economic and political choices there is a *moral dilemma:* on the one hand, serious moral claims have made us expand our demands on medicine to attack age-old threats to human well-being; on the other hand, health care competes with other social benefits, such as education and economic stability. In addition to deciding how much of our resources will be committed to health care, we also must face the fact that *full and complete care cannot be given to everyone* in the society. By what system, then, shall individuals *qualify*? If exclusion is necessary, then by what system shall persons be excluded?

SEVERAL APPROACHES TO DEFINITION

The oldest and most venerable definition of "health" was used by Plato, Aristotle, and Descartes, among others. Their definition, which has found

1. Lead editorial, *Washington Post,* July 18, 1981.

an important place in Western thought, was concerned only with *physical* well-being. Another approach to defining health includes both *physical* and *mental* well-being. The work of Freud, Jung, Adler, and other pioneers in psychoanalysis has contributed to this expansion of the definition of health. Finally, the most inclusive modern definition of health is that of the World Health Organization (WHO), set forth in 1946; this definition includes not only *physical* and *mental* well-being, but *social* well-being as well. The individual's social adjustment is therefore no less important than the person's psychological health. Critics of this third, all-inclusive approach point out that this is precisely the kind of thinking that raises expectations that medicine cannot meet. Critics hold that psychological therapy designed to alter antisocial behavior, for example, is beyond the purview of medical facilities and practitioners as we know them today. Countering this point of view are other commentators who point out that we are only now beginning to understand the full extent of the interconnections between physical, psychological, and social well-being.

This interest in the definition of health is far from purely academic. A controlling definition of health can play a major role in determining the arena and kinds of activity that are deemed legitimate health care *responsibilities*. An example will illustrate the importance of this recent expansion of the definition of health. In 1974, a change was made in the Federal Employees Compensation Act in that federal employees for the first time were allowed to include the treatment given them by psychologists or psychiatrists as legitimate medical costs for reimbursement. Also, the medical reports of psychiatrists and psychologists could support a disability claim (which would enable an employee to continue receiving up to seventy-five percent of his or her salary). Many employers and health insurance plans made similar extensions through the 1970s. These extensions were made possible because a new and expanded definition of "health" readily permitted the inclusion of mental health.

Similarly, it has been argued that toxic substances in the environment are threats to health. Underlying these arguments is the assumption that toxic substances can threaten the physical, mental, *and* social well-being of affected citizens who live near toxic dump sites or nuclear plants that go awry. Some have contended that even before we know precisely how the manufacture, use, and disposal of toxic substances, including nuclear substances, might threaten *physical* health, we can clearly understand how their existence in the environment are a threat to *mental* and *social* well-being. When such threats to human welfare are defined as threats to health, they become the legitimate concern of doctors, nurses, and hospitals—and those affected become eligible for some form of reimbursement of medical costs. As we will see shortly, this sort of development is frequently linked to a broad "right to health" as a freedom *from* such environmental threats to human well-being. This is what we described in the first chapter as a negative right.

THE "RIGHT" TO HEALTH

In 1776, American colonists declared that there were certain "inalienable" rights, among them life, liberty, and the pursuit of happiness. It took a revolutionary war to establish those *declared* rights as *legitimate* rights in a new nation. The evolution of "rights" in Western society is a complex story intertwined with developments in philosophy, politics, and warfare. Some say the story of the evolution of modern rights begins in the West with the Magna Carta, when one segment of the population declared and won certain rights from those above them. John Locke's powerful arguments in the seventeenth century for certain rights and freedoms of the individual provided key philosophical and moral justifications for subsequent legal and political rights that were important to the American and French revolutions.

The evolution of new rights and corresponding obligations for society continued through the nineteenth century. American and European philosophers and reformers claimed, and in some cases won, additional rights. These new rights included rights to work, education, and forms of social security for larger segments of the population. Gradually, these new *social* rights, which extended beyond earlier *political* and *civil* rights, were established as legitimate by certain governments.

A frequent pattern in the evolution of rights has been that a new right will first be claimed as a *moral* right. Eventually, these claims are translated through the legislature or the court system, where precedent-setting legislation or legal opinions are framed. Finally, governmental programs and agencies are established to implement the accepted rights and corresponding obligations.

Claims to rights concerning health have taken two broad forms: a "right to *health*" and a "right to *health care*." The right to health was claimed during the rise of public health programs. During the Industrial Revolution people first became aware that job hazards, sanitation, air and water pollution, and other unwanted side effects of industrialization could have adverse effects on the well-being of individual citizens and demanded protection from such effects of their governments. Likewise, once people understood that germs transmitted disease and could produce widespread epidemics and even pandemics, they began to place claims on their governments to guard against the spread of disease. The governments did respond. For example, there arose new guidelines for workers' safety and programs of mass inoculation. These new kinds of health rights were evolving in the same era that other social rights were being translated into legal rights, such as the rights to education, to decent wages and work hours, and the like.

The claim of a right to health *care* is a more recent claim. This right was asserted when objections arose to various *obstacles* in the paths of many people who sought adequate health care. The obstacles were, in various cases, economic, social, or geographic. Underlying the response to these obstacles was the assumption that everyone ought to have equal access to needed health care. One writer stated it this way: "Every person in the entire resident population should have equal access to health care delivery."[2] That moral claim was expressed by the General Assembly of the United Nations in 1966 as a human right, "the *right* of *everyone* to the enjoyment of the *highest attainable* standard of physical and mental health" (emphasis added). This same document goes on to state that one of the necessary steps to be taken for the realization of this broad "right to health" is through "the creation of conditions which would assure to all [persons] *medical services* and *medical attention* in the event of sickness"[3] (emphases added).

Some industrialized nations have converted these moral claims regarding health and health care into legal rights. The rights now have the force of law and are implemented by government programs and agencies. The British and some other European governments have rather extensive "cradle to grave" health plans. In some of these nations, citizens pay separate taxes, similar to the Social Security tax in the United States, and health care is delivered by practitioners who are employed by the government. In other countries, health care costs are taken out of general tax revenues and practitioners are reimbursed by the government (although not employed by the government). The underlying goal of all such plans is to distribute health care resources more equitably by eliminating various economic, social, or geographic obstacles.

The notion of a right to health care has not been converted into law and practice in the United States as extensively as in other industrial nations. There is no comprehensive health care program, and none has been regarded as having much chance of being adopted in the foreseeable future. National health insurance legislation, which would require our government to guarantee a minimum level of health insurance coverage for *all* citizens, has been introduced but has not progressed very far in the legislative process.

2. Gene Outka, "Social Justice and Equal Access to Health Care," *Journal of Religious Ethics* 2 (Spring 1974): 11 ff.

3. "A Definition of Health," from the Preamble to the Constitution of the World Health Organization Conference, 1946.

Although we have not enacted a comprehensive plan, we have added new groups to the list that already have guaranteed health insurance coverage. For example, from the earliest days of the nation those in military service and veterans of military service have had some form of governmental provision for health care. Both the level of health care and the number of people covered by government guarantee were extended after the two world wars. In 1946, the Hill-Burton Act provided millions, eventually even billions of dollars, for the construction of hospitals. Within the enabling legislation was the provision that the hospitals built with the Hill-Burton money were to provide a "reasonable volume of services . . . to persons unable to pay." That provision was ignored routinely until the 1970s, when a series of lawsuits forced compliance.

The landmark health care legislation affecting access to health care in the United States was enacted in the 1960s—the Medicare and Medicaid legislation. In its Handbook for Implementation of Medicaid Legislation, the (then) Department of Health, Education, and Welfare proclaimed what could be interpreted as acceptance by the government of citizens' rights to health care and the government's corresponding obligation to provide it:

The passage of Title XIX [Medicaid] marks the beginning of a new era in medical care for low-income families. The potential of this new Title can hardly be over-estimated, as *its goal is the assurance of complete, continuous, family-centered medical care of high quality to persons who are unable to pay for it themselves.* [Emphasis added.] This law aims much higher than the mere paying of medical bills, and States, in order to achieve its high purpose, will need to assume responsibility for planning and establishing new systems of high quality medical care, comprehensive in scope and wide in coverage.[4]

While Medicaid was intended to remove economic barriers to health care for low-income people, Medicare was intended to do the same for the elderly and was made part of the Social Security Trust. Today, the reality of these programs is that (1) costs are far beyond what anyone estimated, (2) we are discovering that the affluence of this country is not unlimited and that health care funding must compete with funding for other national programs and priorities, and (3) in spite of increasing expenditures, millions of Americans still are without coverage for health care. In the next chapter we will say more about programs designed to allocate health care resources fairly.

While the *definition* of health and health care is broadening, our health care *practices* really have not kept pace. Public programs in American life

4. Cited in Edward V. Sparer, "The Legal Right to Health Care," *Hastings Center Report,* 6 (October 1976): 43.

still are confined rather closely to the diagnosis and treatment of disease while pressure mounts to use money and personnel for health care activities that go beyond treatment of illness. If an expanded definition of health is accepted to include not only physical well-being, but also mental and social well-being, then new kinds of services will need to be delivered at public expense.

Pressure is mounting also for more government-sponsored activity in preventive medicine and long-term care for the chronically ill. The moral argument is that, since preventive medicine decreases the suffering and increases the health of entire segments of the population, society ought to invest its resources to that end. This reasoning extends even to the need to eradicate a whole range of environmental and social threats to individual and public health.

The best-known mode of health care activity has been, of course, the traditional encounter between an individual doctor and a patient. Now a variety of factors are working against the maintenance of that traditional relationship. Doctors may find themselves having to accept responsibility for the health of others in addition to their fee-paying patients. This does not mean that they simply will be treating some other patients for free—it means that health care practitioners see themselves in expanded roles, protecting the population from environmentally caused diseases, or even from the horror of nuclear accidents or nuclear war.

WEIGHING BENEFITS AGAINST COST

Even in an affluent society, funds are finite. No government-sponsored program can be expanded infinitely, without eventually finding its limit as it begins to compete for money with other programs. *Cost/benefit analysis,* although not a new analytical tool, frequently has been used in recent years by decision-makers when establishing health care laws and programs. Furthermore, the cost/benefit approach is used extensively in formal and informal health care decision-making at the personal, institutional, and societal levels.

Stated most simply, cost/benefit analysis attempts to weigh the costs of one alternative versus the potential benefits of that alternative. Only in a strict sense are costs and benefits measured in dollars, but the use of cost/benefit analysis represents an attempt to *quantify* the consequences of various alternative solutions to a dilemma. For example, consider a study by H. E. Klarman, published in 1965,[5] that calculated the *financial* cost of

5. H. E. Klarman, "Syphilis Control Problems," in *Measuring Benefits of Government Investments,* ed. R. Dorfman, (Washington, D.C.: Brookings Institution, 1965).

eliminating syphilis in the United States. The calculations included medical care expenditures, loss of employment, and other factors. The cost was put at $117.5 million *annually* to eliminate and then continuously prevent syphilis in our society. On the other hand, when projected into the future, the cost of syphilis itself to the society was estimated in the *billions* of dollars. Klarman's cost/benefit analysis of syphilis clearly supported the expenditure to eradicate the disease.

Let us look at another type of cost/benefit problem: how much should society pay to reduce certain *threats* to health? Think about *environmental* effects on health, for example, such as air pollution due to exhaust fumes from automobiles. The *benefit* in this analysis is that, with clean air, the society would spend fewer dollars for medical treatment of certain diseases. The cost could be described in terms of the dollars required to develop and install air pollution control devices on all automobiles. This kind of cost/benefit discussion has been going on in state and federal governments for years. Our society is trying to decide how much it is willing to pay for control devices and for emission control enforcement and, indeed, what level of bad air will be tolerated. As we learn more about the various and new kinds of threats to health, we can identify dozens, even hundreds, of new threats that "ought" to be controlled or eliminated. The cost of dealing with these problems effectively would increase at an alarming rate. Once we recognize that we cannot undertake all programs, then we must face the difficult task of deciding *which ones are most important.* Trade-offs become the name of the game.

Utilitarians generally favor the use of cost/benefit analysis because it provides a rational (or at least a less intuitive and political) basis for finding ways to deliver the greatest good to the greatest number. Deontologists argue that even if cost/benefit analysis can be useful in some domains, there are certain matters, such as health, life, and death, that cannot be converted to monetary values. The critics of cost/benefit analysis are represented clearly in the article by Michael Baram at the end of this chapter. A contrary reading by Gavin Mooney, which could be called utilitarian, is also provided.

Of the many issues we face in this area in the 1980s let us consider more closely two important and illustrative issues—health care of the elderly and environmental threats to health from nuclear and toxic substances.

THE COST OF LIVING LONGER

Place: Washington, D.C.

Time: Sometime in the 1980s

Meeting: Subcommittee on Social Security of the House of Representatives of the U.S. Congress (an imaginary session)

Chairman Steadfast: Ladies and gentlemen, the agenda today includes a discussion of the Medicare program. As you recall, we initiated this program in 1965 under the Social Security Trust Funds to provide medical care to our citizens over age sixty-five. Since then we have expanded benefits, and we have seen a sharp rise in medical costs. Today we are confronted with more eligible recipients than ever before. The projected budget costs for this year will be $35 billion. In our meeting today we have several proposals before us, and I'll ask the sponsors to speak to each of these proposals in turn. First we will hear from our esteemed colleague, Mr. Wainwright.

Congressman Wainwright: Mr. Chairman, I encourage my colleagues to consider the merits of my "back to basics" bill. Mr. Chairman, over the years we have expanded the benefits of Medicare far beyond the original concept of a "safety net for the aged." Now we extend benefits to most any group who can rally a lobbying effort and present an emotional appeal. Take for instance the expenses involved in the end-stage renal disease program. Mr. Chairman, we now spend five percent of the total Medicare budget for this program, and it benefits only two-tenths of one percent of the total eligible Medicare population.

Mr. Chairman, my "back to basics" legislation would even out certain discrepancies and would provide necessary protection from catastrophe, but it would drop all of the frills we now offer. The truth of the matter is that we cannot afford to continue to expand this program. Our monies are not unlimited. We must use the money that we have equitably and fairly for the citizens for whom the Medicare program was intended when it was originally established in 1965.

Congresswoman Fairbrother: Mr. Chairman, I would like the Committee to focus on my bill for what I call a "shared-cost" program. It is clear to me, Mr. Chairman, that when a social benefit is free, it is abused. When the benefit has a cost, it then has a place in the assignment of individual priorities. What I am saying, Mr. Chairman, is that when you pay for it, you will also ask, "Do I really need it?"

My measure would ask that Medicare beneficiaries share more of the cost themselves. Currently, they pay a small monthly premium and are responsible for the first few dollars of the year. With my proposal we will slide the copayments according to the ability to pay. The very poor will be required to pay only a token amount, and the very wealthy will pay up to ninety percent of the total cost of their health care. Mr. Chairman, I propose to you and to this Committee that this is the only fair approach.

Congressman Rotor: Mr. Chairman, my colleagues are confused. I doubt that Mr. Wainwright seriously wants to "pull the plug" on dialysis machines, and surely Ms. Fairbrother can't seriously think that her "Robin Hood" approach is fair.

Mr. Chairman, we made a contract and a promise to all our elderly citizens in 1965 to take care of their health needs. We did not say, "Only some of you," and we did not say "Only if you pay more and more yourselves." For years, the elderly in my district uncomplainingly have paid their wages into the Social Security Trust Fund—*Trust* Fund, Mr. Chairman—fully expecting us to live up to our word as a society, and to keep our promises to them. Now faced with fixed incomes and soaring inflation, these people have a problem not of their own doing. Are we to say, "Sorry, we don't take care of that," or "Sorry, you will have to pay more"? No, Mr. Chairman, my proposal is quite simple. It calls for an increase in the Social Security tax to cover the rising cost of keeping our original promise.

Some Questions to Consider
The above dialogue is hypothetical, but the issue is real and present. If you had to endorse one of the three proposals, which would it be? How would you justify your choice?

On the average, people in our society are living longer than their parents or grandparents. This trend toward longer life is attributable to a number of factors, including the elimination of some communicable diseases, better nutrition, and better health care. The average life expectancy has risen from forty-seven years to seventy-three years within this century. In 1975, only ten percent of the people in the United States were age sixty-five or older; projections show that by the year 2040 twenty-three percent of the population will be sixty-five or older.

The elderly require a disproportionately large share of our health resources. In 1976, the ten percent of the people who were 65 or older required thirty-six percent of our national health expenditure. Put this together with the fact that health care costs in general are rising faster than inflation and you can see that we face a potentially difficult problem that could become a crisis. Could we arrive at a point in the future when there is either an overt or covert policy to withhold certain lifesaving health care resources from citizens older than a certain age?

Many believe that Medicare costs run as high as they do because they subsidize the prevailing private practice of medicine. The program requires no accountability or government intervention, but essentially gives a "blank check" to the patient and the doctor. Dr. David Rogers of the Robert Wood Johnson Foundation summarizes: "Expanded private and public insurance [Medicare and Medicaid] markedly increased the number of dollars flowing to the health sector. However, few foresaw . . . that simply changing the way Americans paid for their care would result in such a phenomenal takeoff in the costs of health care."[6] From 1978 to 1980, the cost of Medicare was estimated to have risen thirty-five percent, to about $35 billion—yet, as critics point out, Medicare today covers only about forty percent of the total health care costs of the elderly. What this means for the individual patient is that he or she is paying more than twice as much out-of-pocket as he or she paid for health care *before* Medicare was established!

6. David E. Rogers, *American Medicine: Challenge for the 1980s*, (Cambridge, Mass.: Ballinger Publishing Co., 1978), p. 31.

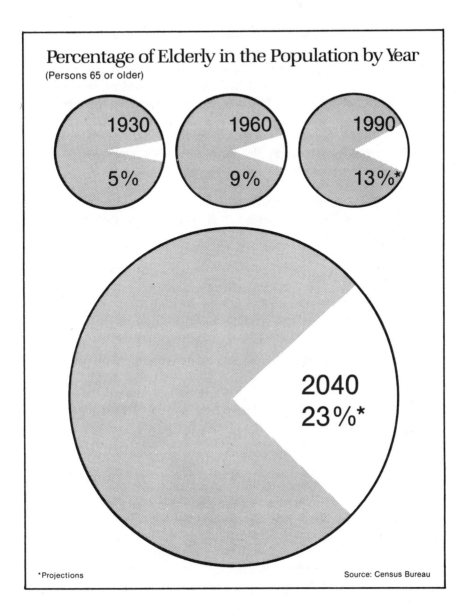

Percentage of Elderly in the Population by Year
(Persons 65 or older)

1930
5%

1960
9%

1990
13%*

2040
23%*

*Projections

Source: Census Bureau

Anne Somers has written: "A decade ago, when many of us thought that American technical and economic sources were unlimited, the Medicare model was tolerated with little criticism. Today, in an era of economic constraints, it is clear that it will have to be reformed or replaced, although no one knows how to do either."[7] If we remember that other new health care programs have been added since Medicare, such as the end-stage renal disease program, it is easy to understand the crisis now faced by public health programs in the aggregate. Year after year, the U.S. Congress searches for answers and debates alternatives.

"What it comes down to is that the gradual aging of Americans, combined with sky-rocketing health costs, forces daily decisions on who shall live and who shall die," according to the president of a major medical center.[8]

HUMAN-MADE DISEASES

In 1979, over fifty environmental groups in California endorsed "The Environmental Bill of Rights."[9] Among the ten "rights" claimed were these three:

- Clear air in urban centers, industrial and agricultural work places, and elsewhere throughout the state;
- Adequate amount of water, unpolluted by toxic wastes or excessive sediments, in streams, rivers, lakes, underground basins, and coastal areas;
- Freedom from involuntary exposure to chemicals, minerals, radioactive substances, and energy forms that are hazardous to health.

The benefits of chemical and nuclear ingenuity are undeniable. They are among the most exciting latter-day outgrowths of the Industrial Revolution. And yet, we share with the earliest participants in the Industrial Revolution the problems that arise from unanticipated costs of technological advance. These costs, we now know, can be very severe, and they can be manifested in unforeseen ways years or even decades after the benefits have been received. Scarcely a week goes by that we do not see a news story referring to "man-made" diseases resulting from environmental pollution or the delayed effects of hazards in the workplace.

Some physicians and many public health experts as well as victims point out that exposure to human-made diseases can require expensive

7. Anne R. Somers, "The 'Geriatric Imperative' and Growing Economic Constraints," *Journal of Medical Education* 55 (February 1980): p. 91.

8. Dr. Thomas Chalmers of New York's Mt. Sinai Medical Center, quoted in the *New York Times,* March 15, 1981.

9. Bill Devall, appendix to book review, *Environmental Ethics* 3 (Spring 1981): 95.

and long-term medical treatment. But the cost of reducing environmental threats to health is high, too. It has been estimated that air and water pollution regulations of the EPA alone will add three-tenths of one percent *annually* to the inflation rate (as measured by the Consumer Price Index between 1970 and 1986). Purely in financial terms, the costs of treating persons with black-lung disease or thousands of citizens who live near polluted environments, such as Love Canal or Three Mile Island, are significant. The cost of enforcing pollution control and safety guidelines on industries such as utilities and chemical manufacturers are high and contribute to inflation. There is no obvious *economic* solution to the dilemma created by greater knowledge of environmental threats to public health and the expanded definition of health that includes threats to physical, mental, and social well-being.

NUCLEAR AND TOXIC ENVIRONMENTAL HAZARDS

ON WEDNESDAY, MARCH 26, 1979, RUMORS BEGAN TO CIRCULATE IN CENTRAL PENNSYLvania about some "trouble" being encountered at the Three Mile Island Nuclear Power Station. At 10:00 A.M. on Friday, March 28, confirmation of serious danger came with the announcement that "an uncontrolled release of radiation gas has occurred."

The words "hydrogen bubble" and "meltdown" were inserted in the world's lexicon with the speed of electronic communications. There was fear but, fortunately, no acute radiation illness victims, no explosion, and no loss of life.

The accident was financially costly. An expense of two billion dollars can be ascribed directly to the accident, a large portion of which has gone to eliminate the threat to citizens' health. This figure includes the costs of replacing the power from other sources, special personnel and technology to handle the accident, reimbursement of expenses incurred by those who evacuated (estimated to be 200,000 residents), and the continuing cost of decontaminating the site and the water in the containment building.

Many people, rightly or wrongly, have paid these bills. The utility company appealed for marked rate increases. Some increases were allowed, but the Public Utility Commission refused to permit the users to take the full burden. The owners of the utility (stockholders) were given no dividends and the value of their stock fell precipitously. State taxpayers took the brunt of state-agency involvement, and federal taxpayers will probably pay to assist in the disposal of the contaminated water.

Some Questions to Consider

In this particular case, a very large sum of money is being spent to contain a human-made threat to health. The amount of money and the effect on the public's imagination of an accident at a nuclear power plant have made the events at

Three Mile Island precedent-setting. Who *should* pay for such threats to health? Should it be:
1. the users of the power from the utility through increased electrical bills?
2. the owners (stockholders) of the utility?
3. all U.S. citizens through federal tax dollars?
4. all residents of the particular state through increased state taxes?
5. all participants in affected insurance plans through increased insurance premiums?
6. a combination of two or more of the above groups?
How would you justify your particular plan for sharing fairly the costs of eliminating environmental threats to health?

We are learning that there are nuclear and chemical substances that may cause cancer, genetic mutation, and other threatening disorders. We do not yet know exactly what level of exposure is required to produce many serious illnesses or under what circumstances the exposure may occur. In order to acquire proof of cause and effect, it may be necessary to monitor effects over a period of decades. Not very much is known about the long-term effects of nuclear and toxic chemical substances. For example, early data suggest (but do not yet prove) that environmental exposure to toxins is increasing the proportion of abnormal sperm in American males, which may in turn contribute to a greater number of fetal deformities. Although there is great temptation to use data like these, many medical researchers warn us against the dangers of using data gathered on small samples and in the short term. Citizens' groups, however, have claimed that fully conclusive scientific evidence is not necessary. It is apparent to these groups already that nuclear and toxic substances are a threat to health and that the government ought to initiate a crash program of research to prove it. In the meantime, they say, the government should control these substances *as if* they were as dangerous as they are suspected of being.

The disposal of nuclear wastes is a perplexing problem. For over thirty-five years now, no solution has been found and nuclear wastes have been accumulating in "temporary" storage facilities around the country. Since the 1920s, researchers have known that low-level exposure to radiation (in the form of X rays) can cause mutations in chromosomal formations. However, not until recently has much serious medical investigation gone into the possible hazards of exposure to various other kinds of low-level radiation. Such studies can require many years to complete. Only now are we beginning to learn the full impact on health of exposure to the *massive* radiation produced at Hiroshima and Nagasaki on August 6 and 9, 1945, the long-range problems of which have included birth defects for succeeding generations and prolonged damage to psychological and social well-being.

Our industries are producing vast quantities of nuclear and chemical waste every day. As a society, sooner or later we must face some decisions. For example, how serious is the threat that we may become ill from the low-level radiation that arises from the presence of nuclear wastes in our environment? Is this a threat that we can or must live with because of a national need for military security or a desire for nonpetroleum sources of energy? Who should pay for the development of technologies that will enable the prudent disposal of nuclear waste—the public's tax dollars? the nuclear industries? Who has the responsibility to monitor possible nuclear threats to health, and who will determine what levels are acceptable?

The disposal of *chemical* wastes poses problems no less difficult than the problem we face with *nuclear* waste. For years, chemical wastes have been disposed of inadequately. Between 1975 and 1978, ninety percent of chemical wastes were disposed of improperly, according to an estimate by the Environmental Protection Agency. Improper disposal means that wastes can reemerge, seen or unseen, in the environment. Later, homes and schools may be built near dangerous dump sites, and residents may find that their plants, animals, and water supplies are contaminated with chemicals long forgotten.

The Love Canal episode in northern New York State focused attention on this problem several years ago. There, chemicals from a long-abandoned dump site seeped above ground and apparently produced skin rashes, nausea, miscarriages, and other illnesses. The surrounding community was thrown into financial chaos and social disruption. During the 1930s and 1940s, the Hooker Chemical Company dumped an estimated 20,000 tons of chemical waste residue in an abandoned canal they owned. In 1953, they sold the site to the Niagara Falls Board of Education for $1, cautioning the board about the possible dangers at the site. Nonetheless, schools and housing developments were built on top of the filled-in canal. As early as the late 1950s, sludge was seeping into basements of the new homes. In 1978, tests were made on the sludge and air in homes and medical tests were performed on residents. By the end of that year almost 240 families had been evacuated. According to the Love Canal Home-owners Association, forty percent of the couples in that relocation have divorced or separated. (Men tended to stay for financial reasons; women tended to flee the site.) In 1980, 700 families in the "outer ring" were moved. Many tests and studies have reported a wide variety of illnesses, birth defects, and miscarriages presumably attributable to the chemical wastes buried under the community. In May 1980, a study was released that reportedly showed chromosomal damage to residents. Although that report was later severely criticized by scientists and discredited in the eyes of many, the initial reaction of the residents was described as "near hysterical" by newspaper accounts. Other studies have been done on the psychological effects of the events at Love Canal. While these studies are inconclusive and some contradict others, the physical, mental, and social well-being of residents has clearly been damaged. As one writer has observed, "Even if the health damage from the chemicals could be definitely ascertained, it would be extremely difficult to sort out which health problems result from [toxic] poisoning and which can be ascribed to emotional stress."[10]

The federal and New York State governments have spent millions of dollars on the health problems at Love Canal. Hooker Chemical has been sued for millions of dollars by public and private groups. The lessons and questions that remain to be understood from the events at Love Canal are still unfolding, but a few are obvious: Should we always wait for "irrefutable" medical evidence of *physical* damage before intervening? How primitive is our knowledge of the toxic causes of cancer, miscarriage, fetal deformities, and chromosomal damage? Should we increase medical research to understand more fully any such possible connections? Are we, as a society, obligated to make certain public policy decisions *before* the full medical data are available? Where do we set a limit on the money we spend to reduce alleged environmental threats to health?

Medical data, even where they are available from long-range studies, can document the costs of our technological "progress," but data cannot resolve the choices that we face as a society. This can be done only by developing some form of moral conviction about costs versus benefits.

David Rutstein, writing an editorial in the *New England Journal of Medicine,* argued that we should intervene to reduce hazards in our environment even before those hazards are fully documented in their effects.

The present intensifying struggle between environmental protection and industrial cost control focuses on the validity of particular risk levels of specific toxic hazards to health. More laboratory and animal experiments and more cost-benefit analyses, valuable as they are, cannot by themselves resolve this conflict. In addition it will be essential to conduct intensive epidemiologic studies of already-exposed populations of harmed and unharmed persons in order to obtain more precise information on the highest tolerable level of risk that does not induce definitive disease. The sooner, the better. In the meantime, when we are faced with an epidemic of serious, clear-cut, man-made disease, will it be too much to ask that, if at all possible, we give the human race the benefit of the doubt?

10. Constance Holden, "Love Canal Residents Under Stress: Psychological Effects May Be Greater Than Physical Harm," *Science* 208 (1980): 1243.

Dr. Rutstein's editorial proposes that human-made disease control is no different from communicable disease control and argues for methods already developed for diagnosis, prevention, treatment, and control of communicable diseases. It goes on to point out that "man-made disease control will impose specific economic costs to eliminate or control a defined hazard."[11]

THE SEARCH FOR A FEASIBLE SOLUTION

We face a series of dilemmas. For each of us individually and for our society collectively, health and the confidence of well-being are those conditions without which all the other benefits of modern life must lose their excitement and flavor. If we are tempted to believe that each person is entitled to health care and protection, we must realize immediately that under the present circumstances we probably cannot afford to provide it for at least many services. Our success in extending longevity has compounded our problem, and our ingenuity in industrialization has produced threats to health that were never envisioned by previous generations. We feel ourselves forced to decide how much health care we shall administer, to whom, and according to what criteria of personal qualification. We make these choices knowing that they will determine who enjoys what level of health and even who shall live and who shall die. Science presses forward to document the hazards, diagnostic techniques, and treatment procedures that might insure greater health for us all—and yet science cannot make the tough calls for us. What we face is not a scientific problem, but a moral question. We are in the position of having to establish public policy in matters of health, life, and death on the basis of our moral *values*. As a society, how much risk are we willing to live with? What segments of the population will receive the benefits and what segments will live with the risks?

DOCTOR STOCKMANN: I tell you the whole situation is a white-sepulcher, spreading poison; it's a menace to the Public Health! All that filth from the tanneries up at Milldale—and you know what a stench there is around there—seeps into the feed pipes of the pump room, and, not only that, but this same poisonous offal seeps out into the beach as well. . . . I was struck by the curious amount of illness among the visitors at the Baths last year—there were several cases of typhoid and gastric fever.

THE MAYOR: A municipal loan will naturally be necessary to clean it up. . . .

11. David D. Rutstein, "Controlling the Communicable and the Man-Made Diseases," *New England Journal of Medicine* 304 (1981): 1423.

ASLAKSEN, CHAIRMAN OF THE HOMEOWNERS' ASSOCIATION: You mean the townspeople would have to pay for it out of their own pockets? I should think the owners of the Bath would be responsible.

THE MAYOR: The owners are not prepared to increase their investment at this time.

ASLAKSEN: But then, damn it, this puts the matter in quite a different light.

THE MAYOR: The worst part of it is, we shall be obliged to close down the Baths for a couple of years.

ASLAKSEN: We could never survive that, Your Honor; we homeowners depend on these visitors—what are we to live on in the meantime? It's downright inexcusable of Dr. Stockman.

THE MAYOR: I've drawn up a short statement on the matter, interpreting the facts from a more rational point of view; I've also indicated ways in which any small defects that might conceivably exist can be taken care of within the scope of the present financial budget.

ASLAKSEN: Everything in moderation!

—Henrik Ibsen,
An Enemy of the People

SELECTED READINGS
Is It Ethical to Place a Monetary Value on Human Life?[12]

Adoption of Cost-Benefit Analysis by Federal Agencies   The continuing efforts of regulatory agencies to balance competing considerations, such as public health and economic feasibility, are beset by a number of special problems. The technical problems include an ever-expanding, but limited and generally inconclusive data base, disagreement among experts on methods for using data, lack of consensus as to findings and their applicability to problems at hand, and unquantifiable attributes. Regulators must also value low probability, high cost events while taking into consideration the diverse and changing values of our pluralistic society. Moreover, an atmosphere of "crisis management" is promoted by statutory time limitations and pressures from various interests.

Mandated by statutes and recent Executive orders to conduct complex "balancing analyses" to reach decisions, regulatory agencies are under considerable pressure to adopt cost-benefit analysis. The use of cost-benefit analysis in regulatory decision processes has been promoted by economic consultants and advisory committees to the agencies drawn from the scientific and engineering communities, including the National Academy of Sciences. In addition, regulated industries have urged agencies to use cost-benefit analysis in considering the economic impacts of regulations. Their efforts include challenging agency actions not prem-

12. Excerpts from Michael S. Baram, "Cost-Benefit Analysis: An Inadequate Basis for Health, Safety, and Environmental Regulatory Decision-Making," *Ecology Law Quarterly* 8 (1980): 473–531 (copyright © 1980, *Ecology Law Quarterly*, reprinted by permission).

ised on cost-benefit analysis in lawsuits, lobbying for amendments to existing statutes to require agencies to engage in cost-benefit analysis, conducting studies demonstrating the inflationary and other adverse economic effects of agency decisionmaking not premised on cost-benefit analysis, and advertising campaigns against regulation conducted without cost-benefit analysis. The public also has become increasingly critical of regulation as a cause of societal and economic ills. . . .

Today, a number of agencies assign monetary values to human life. The Nuclear Regulatory Commission (NRC) uses a value of $1,000 per whole-body rem in its cost-benefit analysis.[a] This figure, multiplied by the number of rems capable of producing different types of deaths, provides dollar values for human life. The Environmental Protection Agency's Office of Radiation Programs establishes its environmental radiation standards at levels that will not cost more than $500,000 for each life to be saved.[b] The Consumer Product Safety Commission uses values ranging from $200,000 to $2,000,000 per life in its analyses.[c]

But the fundamental issue is whether cost-benefit analysis is appropriate at all. Without an answer to this question from Congress or the courts, consideration turns to lesser issues: the proper method of valuation, the substantive basis for valuation (possibly relying on insurance statistics, jury awards, or potential lifetime earnings), and the extent agencies should articulate these issues and provide procedures for participation in the valuation process.

To date, agencies have expressed surprisingly little concern about these unresolved problems associated with cost-benefit analysis. Although officials deny valuing unquantifiable factors, these valuations are implicit in any cost-benefit based policy decision involving risks to human life. Responsible decisionmaking demands that implicit valuations be acknowledged and addressed explicitly.

The Chronic Problem of the Discount Rate for Valuing Future Benefits and Costs in Present Analyses   The discount rate is yet another controversial issue afflicting cost-benefit analysis. Stokey and Zeckhauser note that "no observed rate of return

a. 10 C.F.R. [Code of Federal Regulations] pt. 50 app. I (1979).

b. Interview with Dr. William Rowe, Chief, Radiation Program Office, EPA, in Washington, D.C. (1977). Dr. Rowe stated that EPA would not propose a radiation standard for the uranium fuel cycle that would cost more than $500,000 to save an additional, unspecified human life in the general population; it would save a life if the cost were less than $100,000. For costs in between, EPA makes an ad hoc determination.

c. See B. Shimmei, "Consumer Product Safety Commission: Risk Management Regulation and the Use of Cost-Benefit Analysis" (May 1978) (unpublished draft for M. Baram project on Federal Regulation and Risk Management, based in part on extensive interviews with CPSC personnel). For an extensive Department of Transportation report setting values for human life, see National Highway Traffic Safety Administration, U.S. Department of Transportation, *Societal Costs of Motor Vehicle Accidents* (December 1976). This work and its periodic revisions are frequently consulted and cited with respect to monetary valuation of human life and health. The National Bureau of Standards, in its studies to find technical solutions to problems of flammable fabrics and other consumer hazards for regulatory agencies such as the Consumer Product Safety Commission (CPSC), has used a value of $300,000 per life in arriving at its recommendations. See U.S. National Bureau of Standards, *Preliminary Report on Evaluating Alternatives for Reducing Upholstered Furniture Fire Losses* 13 (November 1977) (NBSIR–77–1381).

can provide an accurate reading of the intertemporal preferences of the society as a whole. . . . [T]he choice of a discount rate should be used deliberately to apportion costs and benefits among income groups and . . . generations, according to the values held by society."[d] Congress and the courts, however, have not decided upon a standard discount rate to establish the present value for future dollar levels of predicted attributes, such as future ecological dislocation, mutagenic effects on future generations, and other long-term consequences of actions taken by regulatory agencies.

Absent a societal decision on the appropriate discount rate, the task of establishing a present value for the future effects of agency decisions falls upon the individual analyst. This has resulted in arbitrary, inconsistent determinations in many cost-benefit analysis decisions. For instance, agency analysts have not agreed on a discount rate for the long-term carcinogenic and mutagenic effects of radioactive isotopes and toxic chemicals. Suggested rates for the future costs of cancer and other diseases range from six to ten percent, without any notable underlying rationale.[e] Analysts seem to be feeling their way toward some sign of societal acquiescence on a discount rate for long-term health and environmental attributes.

But focusing on the search for the societally acceptable number for discounting the future clouds the larger issue: whether using these economic principles in contemporary decisionmaking adequately ensures the desirable quality of life and health for future generations. Ultimately, the discount rate issue is an ethical problem that transcends economic and legal perspectives.

Improper Distribution of Costs and Benefits   Every regulatory decision on health, safety, or environmental problems results in costs and benefits that will be distributed in some pattern across different population sectors, and in many cases, over several generations. For example, a decision to allow the commercial distribution of a toxic substance may result in economic benefits to the industrial users, their shareholders and employees, and consumers. It may also result, however, in adverse health effects and property damage to plant employees and those living near the plant. In addition, future generations may suffer mutagenic health effects or the depletion or pollution of natural resources. . . .

Environmental Protection Agency   Statutory vagueness has caused considerable uncertainty as to whether EPA must perform cost-benefit analysis or any other form of balancing when regulating air, water, and radiation. Ordinarily, this uncertainty is resolved under particular statutory provisions only after EPA has acted, when regulated industries bring lawsuits contending that the agency should have relied on a more formal cost-benefit analysis approach. In such cases,

---

d. E. Stokey and R. Zeckhauser, *A Primer for Policy Analysis* (1978), p. 173. See R. Campbell, *Food Safety Regulation 19* (AEI-Hoover Study 12, August 1974).

e. D. Rice and T. Hodgson, "Social and Economic Implications of Cancer in the United States" (June 1978) (report presented by statisticians and economists at the National Center for Health Statistics, U.S. Department of Health, Education, and Welfare to Expert Committee on Cancer Statistics of the World Health Organization and the International Agency for Research on Cancer at Madrid, Spain), p. 13.

earlier clarification of congressional intent would improve EPA's ability to meet its statutory obligations within mandated time periods.

The Clean Air Act, for example, precludes consideration of economic cost in setting standards for hazardous air pollutants, regulating most fuel additives, and establishing national primary and secondary ambient air standards. In other areas of decisionmaking, however, the statute allows consideration of economic costs.

Authority to use cost-benefit analysis in regulating pesticides is more clearly defined. The Federal Environmental Pesticide Control Act of 1972 requires the registration of pesticides. Before approving a registration request, EPA must determine that the pesticide "will perform its intended function without unreasonable adverse effects on the environment."[f] These are cost-benefit based determinations because "unreasonable adverse effects on the environment" is defined as "any unreasonable risk to man or the environment, taking into account the economic, social, and environmental costs and benefits of the use of any pesticide."

The Toxic Substances Control Act permits EPA to take a balancing approach to the regulation of toxic chemical substances and mixtures by authorizing regulation when there is a reasonable basis to conclude that unregulated manufacturing, distribution, or other activity involving a chemical may "present an unreasonable risk of injury to health or the environment."[g] In promulgating a rule under this section, EPA must develop findings on four factors:

(A) the effects of such substance or mixture on health and the magnitude of the exposure of human beings to such substance or mixture,

(B) the effects of such substance or mixture on the environment and the magnitude of the exposure of the environment to such substance or mixture,

(C) the benefits of such substance or mixture for various uses and the availability of substitutes for such uses, and

(D) the reasonably ascertainable economic consequences of the rule, after consideration of the effect on the national economy, small business, technological innovation, the environment, and public health.

Based on this analysis of costs and benefits, EPA must adopt the "least burdensome" requirements necessary to protect against the risk of injury from the regulated substance. . . .

Cost-Benefit Analysis v. Cost-Effectiveness Analysis   Cost-benefit analysis is an unacceptable basis for governmental decisionmaking on persistent health, safety, and environmental problems. It is a simplistic tool that reduces concern for the individual to a monetized balancing. Worse, it has become a self-serving numbers game obscuring arbitrary and subjective values and assumptions, while impeding real progress toward our espoused health, safety, and environmental objectives.

Solutions to societal problems, such as nuclear reactor safety and human ex-

---

f. Environmental Pesticide Act § 3(c)(5)(C), 7 U.S.C. [United States Code] § 136a(c)(5)(C).

g. 15 U.S.C. § 2605(a)(Supp. I 1977). For a general discussion of environmental risks presented by toxic chemicals, see Page,"A Generic View of Toxic Chemicals and Similar Risks," *Ecology Law Quarterly* 7 (1978): 207.

posure to chemical carcinogens, require consideration of humanistic and environmental principles. Consideration of these principles is incompatible with a regulatory decisionmaking process in which economic factors play a dominant role. . . .

The use of cost-benefit analysis also raises larger ethical questions. Our constitutional framework for governmental decisionmaking involves balancing many factors. It does not mandate the use of an economic framework, and indeed establishes a framework for decisionmaking, which ensures that no single factor such as economics will dominate. The varied and often conflicting needs and desires of many segments of our society must be weighed against fundamental individual rights in order to establish ultimate societal values and reach an optimal governmental choice. This process is subverted when cost-benefit analysis is the basis of decisionmaking. An economic framework for making societal choices stresses only factors that are monetizable over a short period of time. Therefore, the use of cost-benefit analysis to determine our policies on such issues as radioactive waste disposal or access for the handicapped to public transportation systems inevitably leads to different results than those obtained by an analysis emphasizing long-term needs or individual welfare.

Public recognition of the ethical implications of governmental adoption of an economic framework for decisionmaking has been woefully insufficient. Responsibility for articulating public values lies with Congress. . . .

A Final Perspective   The cost-benefit techniques used today are the analytical descendants of Jeremy Bentham's proposals for reforming legal decisionmaking through the use of "felicific calculus." Much of the philosophical and humanistic criticism of the Bentham approach remains valid today and is reinforced by constitutional principles that reflect a more holistic approach to governance in a pluralistic society and limit the uses of economic analysis in decisionmaking. In essence, the Constitution does not require that governmental decisionmaking be premised on simplistic economic analyses.

Nevertheless, a strong argument can be made that providing the greatest good for the greatest number remains one of the essential purposes of government, and that cost-benefit analysis represents a potentially workable method to reach this objective. The Executive and its agencies have the responsibility to manage the federal enterprise rationally in order to achieve optimal use of our limited resources and optimal protection of our diverse interests. If cost-benefit analysis continues as a basis for regulatory agency decisionmaking, it must be accompanied by meaningful public participation, diligent congressional, executive, and judicial supervision, and agency "best efforts" to structure their discretion to meet the issues presented by this economic approach to the problems of health, safety, and environmental protection.

Is It Ethical *Not* to Use Cost-Benefit Analysis?[13]

To underline the need for greater understanding by health service decision makers of the relationship between cost-benefit analysis and medical ethics it is necessary

13. Excerpts from Gavin H. Mooney, "Cost-Benefit Analysis and Medical Ethics," *Journal of Medical Ethics* 6 (December 1980): 177–79.

to look no further than a sample of quotations from an article entitled 'Choosing Priorities' by Muir Gray[a] which was published in this journal. He writes: 'The strength of cost-benefit analysis, or any other concept is a function of its weakest point, which is that it attempts to place a monetary value on human life', which he claims 'is not like the value of sheet steel, ball bearings, or any of the other commodities for which cost-benefit analysis is usually employed. It cannot be expressed in monetary terms.' He continues that 'cost-benefit analysis does not provide the decision maker with incontrovertible criteria' and maintains that the choice between treating different groups of patients 'has to be made on ethical, not on financial grounds'.

Now these quotes contain some interesting misconceptions about the use and usefulness of cost-benefit analysis in health care. In particular it is claimed explicitly that a money price cannot be attached to human life and implicitly that somebody, somewhere, has suggested that cost-benefit analysis can 'provide the decision maker with incontrovertible criteria'. On the latter point it would be most valuable if a source could have been quoted to substantiate this purported claim for cost-benefit analysis in health care; it is extremely doubtful if any health care cost-benefit analyst would make any claims for his tools beyond that of decision-*aiding*.

Certainly it is difficult to believe that any economist would argue that cost-benefit analysis provides 'incontrovertible criteria'. As three leading exponents of such analyses have written recently:[b] 'there can be no uniquely "proper" way to do cost-benefit analysis . . . The failure of cost-benefit analysis to give a unique answer to the question of whether a scheme is desirable is in no way a criticism of the technique itself. On the contrary, whenever there is dispute as to the *moral* (emphasis added) notions to be used in evaluating a scheme, it is likely that the results of a cost-benefit study will vary according to which of the opposing value systems is adopted.'

There is however *prima facie* a more substantial criticism contained in the charge that life cannot be valued. There is no market for life in the way that there is for commodities such as academic journals or lawnmowers. At first sight it might appear that life insurance is in some way relevant to life valuation but, insofar as it is, it is rather distant. (Thus the sum insured payable on a man's death might be taken at best to be the value *he* perceives his wife and family place on his life.) But the fact that there is no market for life does not mean it has no monetary value. There is no market for clean air—but do we not value clean air? Are we not prepared to pay for a cleaner environment? And in being prepared to pay are we not thereby placing a monetary value on clean air?

Clearly most of us value life. Yet to pose the questions; at what price do you value your life or your spouse's life or your friend's life? or what would you be prepared to pay to avoid death? is almost meaningless and insofar as such questions do convey any meaning they are well nigh impossible to answer.

a. J. A. Muir Gray, "Choosing Priorities," *Journal of Medical Ethics* 5 (1979): 73–75.

b. C. Nash, D. Pearce, and J. Stanley, "An Evaluation of Cost-Benefit Analysis Criteria," *Scottish Journal of Political Economy* 22 (1975): 121–34.

Does it thereby follow that the value of life is infinite—or that it is impossible to measure satisfactorily? Let us examine these two different questions.

If the value of life were infinite what would our day to day world look like? Certainly it would be very different from what it currently is. The bedroom in which we waken, as well as all the rest of our home, would be safeguarded against *all* possible risk from storms, flood, fire, etc. It is difficult to see how we could convey ourselves to work since there are clearly risks involved whether we walk, drive, cycle or travel by bus or train. We would certainly not indulge in any sporting activity or indeed any other activity in which any mortality risk was involved—if we valued life infinitely. Indeed it is difficult to believe that such an existence would warrant the title life.

Here in essence lies the key to the issue. In practice we are prepared to trade-off a higher risk of death than is strictly necessary in order to enjoy some of the good things of life. We do what amounts to our own personal 'cost-benefit analysis'—not in terms of our lives *per se* but in terms of risk of death. We may not be as well informed about such risks as we might be; nonetheless in deciding how to allocate our income and time we attempt to balance risk against benefits. Sometimes it is money directly that is involved—we buy cheaper but less safe cars; but often other things are entailed—we cross the road by the quicker and more dangerous surface route rather than the longer but safer underpass.

In making such trade-offs they imply first of all a monetary value for risk reduction and secondly a value of life. (Thus if a thousand people are each prepared to pay £100 to reduce their risk of death from 2 in 1000 to 1 in 1000, then the value of the statistical life involved is £100,000.)

A simple example will serve to indicate how this type of process can occur in public policy. Sinclair[c] has shown that the decision to introduce legislation to make cabs on tractors compulsory, thereby reducing mortality risk for tractor drivers in roll over accidents and saving an estimated 200 lives, was achieved at a cost of £20 million, implying that tractor drivers' lives were valued at *at least* £100,000 each. On the other hand Gould[d] indicates that the decision by the Government in 1971 not to introduce child proofing of drug containers to reduce the associated risks for children implied a value of a child's life of less than £1000.

Just as individuals, faced with finite incomes and finite time, *have* to place a finite value on life (or more accurately risk of death) so the health service faced with finite resources *has* to place a value on life. Every decision on resource allocation in the health sector involves a judgement on whether it is worth paying X to achieve Y. If the decision is yes, then Y is being valued at at least X; if the decision is no then Y is being valued at less than X.

Whether it is possible to measure the value of life in some systematic fashion is more problematic. Certainly various attempts have been made to do so.[e] None is wholly satisfactory as yet. What is almost certainly true however is that the value of life (or reduced risk of death) is likely to vary according to a number of factors

c. C. Sinclair, "Costing the Hazards of Technology," *New Scientist,* October 16, 1969, pp. 120–22.

d. D. Gould, "A Groundling's Notebook," *New Scientist,* July 22, 1971, p. 217.

e. G. H. Mooney, *The Valuation of Human Life* (London: Macmillan, 1977).

eg the characteristics of the individual at risk—age, for example; the circumstances of the risk; the level of the risk; and so on. It is therefore unlikely that there is a single uniquely correct value of life but rather a series of values reflecting the fact that life is not a homogeneous 'commodity'.

Further, insofar as we as individuals or the health service as a corporate body are concerned with the issue of valuation of life it is seldom in the context of life versus death. (It should be noted here that in the health service context it is at a *resource planning* level that the interest of cost-benefit analysts lies, not individual patient management. Thus the issue is how much dialysis not whether Mrs Jones or Mr Brown should be dialysed.) The relevant question to be posed is: what are we (and others) prepared to pay to reduce the risk of death from some level much less than one to an even lower level? This is the question we face, frequently subconsciously, in going about our everyday business and it is consequently this question which carries most relevance and meaning in life valuation.

However what is possible is to disentangle the implied values of life contained in decisions on resource allocation. By making such implied values explicit we can reveal inconsistencies in such decision making. Thus in the interests of consistency we would want to spend the same amount on saving similar lives. But in addition we can call on both distributive justice and efficiency to justify such an analysis. It would be inequitable to spend £500,000 to save a life in the context of one form of treatment and refuse to spend £5000 in another (assuming similar lives were involved). Clearly such a disparity in implied values would also be inefficient since a shift of resources from the former policy to the latter would result overall in a greater number of lives being saved. It is here that cost-benefit analysis comes into its own since it is the purpose of cost-benefit analysis to assist in achieving a more efficient use of resources.

It is by compelling decision makers in health care to face up to these issues explicitly that economics and economists can make a contribution to health care planning. Muir Gray[f] suggests that 'the ethical concept which is most relevant to the choosing of priorities is that of distributive justice' and that 'the most important criterion should be the effectiveness of the services which are under consideration.' Certainly distributive justice (or equity) is important but as indicated equally so is efficiency. Too often the medical profession would wish to ignore questions of efficiency and particularly the resource consequences of their decisions. Sometimes the medic is the mirror image of Wilde's cynic, he knows the value of everything and the price of nothing. The strength of cost-benefit analysis, not its weakness as Muir Gray would have it, lies in its ability to force consideration of the issue of placing values on health outcomes and thereby to promote the cause of efficiency in health care. It is not a question of ethics *or* economics. Without a wider use of economics in health care inefficiencies will abound and decisions will be made less explicitly and hence less rationally than is desirable: we will go on spending large sums to save life in one way when similar lives but in greater number could be saved in another way. The price of inefficiency, inexplicitness and irrationality in health care is paid in death and sickness. Is *that* ethical?

f. See note a, above.

ANNOTATED BIBLIOGRAPHY
Books and Articles

Bayles, Michael D. "National Health Insurance and Non-Covered Services." *Journal of Health Politics, Policy and Law* 2 (1977): 335–48. A wide-ranging, philosophical exploration of the justification and justice of various schemes of national health insurance.

Dubos, Rene. *Mirage of Health*. New York: Harper & Row, 1959. A scientist sympathetic to the WHO definition of health writes broadly about the nature of health and disease.

Gert, Bernard, and Charles Culver. *Philosophy in Medicine*. New York: Oxford University Press, 1982. A philosopher and psychiatrist write about several philosophical problems about medical practice, including the nature of disease. Both moral and conceptual problems are addressed.

Anthologies

Beauchamp, Tom L., and LeRoy Walters, eds. *Contemporary Issues in Bioethics*. 2nd ed. Belmont, Calif.: Wadsworth Publishing Company, 1982. Chaps. 2, 9, 10. Many of the most important essays on the subjects addressed in this chapter are found in this volume, including essays that have become classics on the subject.

Bunker, John P., Benjamin A. Barnes, and Frederick Mosteller, eds. *Costs, Risks, and Benefits of Surgery*. New York: Oxford University Press, 1977. A widely acclaimed volume on this specific subject.

Journal of Medicine and Philosophy. Vol. 1 (1976), special issue on "Concepts of Health and Disease." Vol. 2 (1977), special issue on "Mental Health." Vol. 4 (1979), special issue on the "Right to Health Care." Vol. 5 (1980), special issue on "Social and Cultural Perspectives on Disease." These four special issues of this major journal contain a wealth of interdisciplinary reflection on the above-mentioned special topics.

Articles from the *Encyclopedia of Bioethics*

Health and Disease
  I. History of the Concepts *Guenter B. Risse*
  II. Religious Concepts *Frank De Graeve*
  III. A Sociological and Action Perspective *Talcott Parsons*
  IV. Philosophical Perspectives *H. Tristram Engelhardt, Jr.*
Health Policy
  I. Evolution of Health Policy *Stephen P. Strickland*
  II. Health Policy in International Perspectives *Odin W. Anderson*
Public Health *Harold Fruchtbaum*

Literature

Ibsen, Henrik. *An Enemy of the People*. In *Eleven Plays of Henrik Ibsen*. New York: Modern Library, n.d. Dr. Thomas Stockman, the Medical Officer of the Municipal Baths, discovers a threat to the health of the town from contamination by the town's industries. Ibsen's play explores the economic consequences of his discovery and the reactions of the town's businessmen and populace. Pushed to extremes, he becomes the town's moral crusader for an ideal health environment.

Gunn, James. "Medic" (originally "Not So Great an Enemy," 1957, and a part of the *Immortals,* 1962). In *Some Dreams are Nightmares.* New York: Charles Scribner's, 1973. A futuristic short story of a time when 52.5 percent of the national income goes for health care in the form of insurance coverage, "Medic" compares the treatment received by those insured with that received by the noninsured. More intriguing for its imaginative ideas than its satisfactory ending.

Audio/Visual

"A Plague on Our Children." "NOVA" series, two 57-minute films or videotapes. Sale or rental, Time/Life Video, 100 Eisenhower Drive, Paramus, N.J., 07652. Part I, "Dioxins," explores the effects of herbicides on health and as a possible mutagen. Part II, "PCBs," investigates the problems of inadequate toxic waste disposal and its possible short-term and long-term impact on health.

7

HEALTH CARE . . . FOR WHOM?

The following article, which originally appeared in the *Wall Street Journal,* serves as the introductory case in this chapter. It also serves as a transition from the subjects in chapter 6, for it too deals with the crucial problem of the just distribution of health care resources.

NEW YORK—IT WAS A REAL-LIFE EPISODE WITH ELEMENTS WORTHY OF A TELEVISION drama:

A young woman is rushed to an emergency room with internal bleeding. An astute piece of medical detective work reveals that she has a rare blood disorder. While medical teams labor heroically to help her, the nation is scoured for supplies of a rare drug that she must have.

It's touch and go, but after 25 days the patient leaves the hospital alive and well. Later comes the part that likely wouldn't get mentioned in the TV treatment: the cost. The hospital's bill in this case totaled a dazzling $358,942.88, of which the patient's only out-of-pocket cost was $17.60, for telephone calls!

Therein lies a cautionary tale about rising American health costs. Factor VIII inhibition, the woman's ailment, admittedly is unusual; physicians say that fewer than 50 cases like hers are found in the medical literature (and the drug to combat it accounted for $333,858 of the woman's bill). A cursory check by the Health Insurance Association suggests that this may be the largest bill ever run up by a patient for a single illness.

But the Columbia Presbyterian Hospital in Manhattan paid the tab. There were difficult decisions during the illness about whether to use certain procedures and bits of technology whose cost-effectiveness was questionable. And now the complex methods by which the bill was paid are going to raise hospital bills for thousands of other patients and their health-insurance carriers.

What is the alternative? To let a patient die?[1]

1. *Wall Street Journal,* December 10, 1981.

Some Questions to Consider
1. Did the doctors do the right thing with their all-out effort to save this young woman's life, regardless of cost or who she was?
2. Should other considerations have influenced their decision, such as the size of the bill, who would pay for it, how much it would drive up the premiums of others if an insurance company paid the bill (or taxes if Medicaid covered costs)?
3. If she had been in her seventies with no family, would it be harder to justify such an all-out effort?
4. What kind of a society do you want to live in—one that uses available health care resources for each and every person no matter what the effect on total health care costs and the economy, or one that conditions access to health care on the ability to pay, on proximity to major medical centers, on "social worth" of the potential patient, or on some other factor?

In legislation and social organizations, proceed on the principle that invalids, meaning persons that cannot keep themselves alive by their own activities, cannot, beyond reason, expect to be kept alive by the activity of others. There is a point at which the most energetic policeman or doctor, when called upon to deal with an apparently drowned person, gives up artificial respiration, although it is never possible to declare with certainty, at any point short of decomposition, that another five minutes of the exercise would not effect resuscitation. The theory that every individual alive is of infinite value is legislatively impracticable. No doubt the higher the life we secure to the individual by wise social legislation, the greater his value to the community, and the more pains we shall take to pull him through any temporary danger or disablement. But the man who costs more than he is worth is doomed by sound hygiene as inexorably as by sound economics.

—George Bernard Shaw,
preface to *The Doctor's Dilemma*

In spite of the fact that modern societies spend elaborate sums on health, and although health care costs in the United States have been rising at a rate second only to the increase in the cost of oil, the benefits of health care remain unevenly distributed. In 1980, we spent an estimated $245 *billion* on health care, a figure that breaks down to more than $1000 for every U.S. citizen. Despite this enormous investment, all Americans do not share the benefits of our present health care system equitably. Numerous studies reveal the same picture over and over: the poor, nonwhite, elderly, and those who live in urban ghettos or remote rural areas are in much worse health and receive far fewer benefits from our present health care system than do most other Americans. While many of the programs initated in the 1960s have changed this picture somewhat, the basic pattern of distribution remains.

One Institute of Medicine study[2] of poor children in our nation's capital showed that twenty-five percent of those between the ages of six months and two years had anemia. About twenty percent had overt middle ear disease, and seven percent had hearing losses in the speech frequency serious enough to limit learning. Studies of those in rural areas, of the elderly in all areas, and of blacks, Mexican-Americans, and other non-white minorities reveal similar statistics. Millions of Americans have the same level of health as "primitive" persons in underdeveloped nations in Africa and Asia—in spite of our enormous investment and seemingly out-of-control health care costs.

Some modern countries, notably some European nations and Canada, long ago established government health care systems. In the United States, we have accumulated a *mixed, free-market system* of health care delivery. It is free-market in that the primary mode of health care delivery is a fee-for-service (FFS), private relationship between an individual patient and doctor, but it is mixed in that some groups receive third-party subsidies. The two biggest, and most expensive, government programs are Medicare and Medicaid. Critics say that our mixed system leads to cases such as the one with which this chapter began: millions of Americans receive practically no health care, while others who happen to be covered by our patchwork system of subsidization may receive the most sophisticated and expensive medical care available anywhere in the world. Insurance premiums or taxes must cover such costs.

The rules for the distribution of health care resources in any country are related to its whole system of values. Specifically, its system to distribute health care in a "fair" way is linked to its overt or covert concept of distributive justice. What concept of distributive justice does our society rely upon? This is a large question, which can be answered in part by a close examination of our system of distributing health care.

In recent years, our mixed, free-market system has been questioned. Some argue in its defense; others argue that it is not adequate for the present or the future. Those who defend it say that it needs more freedom and less regulation and that competition will bring about "proper" distribution. Others argue that the government is inexorably involved in the delivery of health care and that its involvement must be more enlightened, more intentional, and better planned. They also question whether free-market enterprise, with its emphasis on the profit motive, is the best mode

2. Cited in David E. Rogers, *American Medicine: Challenges for the 1980s* (Cambridge, Mass.: Ballinger Publishing Co., 1978), p. 34.

of delivery of health care. The following excerpts from a "MacNeil-Lehrer Report" aired on the Public Broadcasting System (PBS) in 1981 demonstrate the shape of public deliberation occurring in our society. The three speakers quoted are Mr. Michael Bromberg, Executive Director, Federation of American Hospitals, Arnold Relman, M.D., editor of the *New England Journal of Medicine,* and Robert MacNeil, one of the hosts of the program.

Mr. Bromberg:

Under a market system you have to justify it [rising health costs] to the consumers. Now let me give you a few examples of what I mean. We endorsed the Planning Act in 1974. We endorsed its expansion. We've steadily endorsed it, and this year we turned around and said it's time to phase out the Federal Health Planning Act . . . The reason for it is a waste of money. There are literally thousands of people working on this federally-paid-for system which is not producing results. It is producing burden and cost. I had a situation last year where a hospital in Kentucky wanted to put a new carpet in the hospital, and because it was going to cost more than $100,000, they spent 12 months with lawyers, accountants and experts testifying, and were finally turned down by the so-called planners on the ground that the carpet wasn't frayed enough. Other examples about surfacing parking lots or replacing a small machine. Planning was meant to tackle big issues like, should we build a new hospital? And we've got thousands of people spending time harassing people. Now, on the big ticket items, I'm not saying we shouldn't have a planning system; I'm saying that we don't need a federally-funded, federally-mandated system. Let the States do it, and if competition works, maybe we don't need it at all. Peer review is another example. I think peer review's the key to the—is really the critical answer. And I don't think we are going to get health costs under control in this country until we get the doctors to really get serious about peer review. But you are never going to do that through the government. . . . Competition invokes pressure from consumers. . . .

Mr. MacNeil:

Whatever it might do to costs, some experts are concerned about the quality and availability of health care under a competitive system. One such person is Dr. Arnold Relman, Editor of the *New England Journal of Medicine.* Dr. Relman is with us in the studios of Public Television Station WGBH in Boston. Dr. Relman, what's wrong, in your view, with a competitive system for medicine?

Dr. Relman:

Well, Robert, I think that competition in general is a good idea when it can contribute to keeping costs down and maintaining the quality and accessibility of care. The question is, will competition by itself, in a free market, do that? I have some reservations about it. I used to be more enthusiastic about this idea, and I think along with many other doctors around the country now, have begun to have some reservations. In the first place, no competitive system is going to eliminate regulations. And I think it is a mistake to imagine that we won't need lots of regulation from the federal government to assure quality of care, maintenance of standards, accessibility of care, and so on. In the second place, the emphasis in competition is on price competition, using the profit motive to facilitate the process. And I have very serious reservations about the role of profit motive for providing health care.

Mr. McNeil:

What are those?

Dr. Relman:

Well, in the first place, I don't think that health care is a commodity like a pair of shoes or a refrigerator that can be sold . . . I don't think that we have a free market and will never have a free market in the economists' sense for health care. Health care is, in a certain sense, a right. Not entirely, but clearly it's different from many other things that are bought and sold. And in the second place, the profit motive may distort the way health care is delivered. It may influence the overuse of technology; it may cause fragmentation of care. It may cause a skimming of the profitable patients by the profit-making providers, leaving the expensive, unprofitable patients to the nonprofits.[3]

HOW WE GOT HERE

Commentators have identified several factors that have contributed to the situation in which the costs of health care are becoming burdensome even as its benefits remain unevenly distributed. For example, reimbursement for medical services by private insurance companies and government programs is an important factor. Private insurance plans began in the Great Depression and grew dramatically after World War II, so that today most American workers have some form of health insurance coverage. However, as we all know, these private health insurance companies do not cover anyone who cannot pay the premiums. Furthermore, they tend to reimburse costs for treating acute illness, but do not pay for outpatient care or preventive care.

Historically, the *government* has reimbursed certain segments of the population for their health care. Those in military service were the first to receive such subsidies, then veterans, American Indians, the mentally ill, those with contagious diseases, and some of the poor through emergency-room care in local hospitals that receive government funding. Social Security legislation in the 1930s included many more citizens, but not all. In the 1960s, Medicare, providing aid to the elderly, and Medicaid, providing aid to those on welfare, greatly expanded the number of recipients and the level of governmental subsidy. Today, as we have seen, most Ameri-

3. "Competitive Medicine," transcript from "The MacNeil-Lehrer Report," WNET, New York, July 31, 1981 (copyright 1981 by Educational Broadcasting Corporation and GWETA).

cans receive some form of reimbursement for health care costs, but this coverage is not keeping up with the costs incurred by those who are covered. At the same time, *millions* of Americans still have *no coverage at all.* National health insurance plans, proposed and debated in the 1960s and 1970s to provide some health care coverage for *all* Americans, are receiving very little attention today. The political trend of the 1980s seems to be a reversal of the previous trend to extend governmental coverage to more and more people. Current private and governmental insurance coverage plans in the United States reinforce the open-market system for access to health care resources. Some observers claim that society has further obligations than reinforcing the open market and that citizens have rights that are being violated by this system. One commentator, Dan Beauchamp, has written:

> The preponderance of our public policy for health continues to define health care as a consumption good to be allocated primarily by private decisions and markets, and only interferes . . . to subsidize, supplement or extend the market system where private decisions result in sufficient imperfections or inequity to be of public concern. Medicare and Medicaid are examples. . . .
> Market justice is a pervasive ideology protecting the most powerful. . . . [But] public health should advocate a "counter-ethic" for protecting the public's health, one articulated in a different tradition of justice.[4]

Critics also point out that the American system of health care invests itself heavily in the treatment of acute disease while giving too little attention to *preventive* medicine and *long-term* care. The opening case in this chapter, in which $333,858 was spent on a single drug therapy, reinforces their argument. They say that the drama, money, and prestige of the medical profession are associated with the treatment of life-threatening situations and that this atmosphere is at the heart of the problem. When the health practitioner, using a full arsenal of sophisticated and costly machines and procedures, literally saves a person's life from immediate threats, the patient and family are effusively grateful. This kind of activity fulfills the dramatic image of the deliverer of "heroic medicine," say the critics. Preventive medicine and long-term care simply are less glamorous, and also less rewarding financially.

According to this analysis, the high reward attached to providing care for acute illness has resulted in an oversupply of specialists in the medical profession. Statistics do show that in countries where there are more physicians who specialize in some kind of surgery there are in fact more surgical operations. Where surgery is performed frequently, health care costs are higher. One statistic cited in this discussion is that in the United

---

4. Dan E. Beauchamp, "Public Health as Social Justice," *Inquiry*, March 1976, pp. 4–6.

States twenty-five percent of the total number of physicians are in surgical specialties, compared with thirteen percent in England and Wales and that, proportionately, there are about twice as many operations in the United States.

Next we will consider some actual and proposed solutions to the problems discussed in this and the preceding chapter—then try to discover their underlying moral assumptions.

WHERE DO WE GO FROM HERE?

If it is true that our problem with "distributive justice" in the delivery of health care stems from the fee-for-service (FFS) model for bringing a doctor together with a patient, then we ought to be examining some alternatives to that model. One such alternative to FFS has been "health maintenance organizations" (HMOs). An HMO is a cooperative plan created voluntarily to serve a specific group of people who pay an annual fee for access to a certain medical care facility and its professional staff. Among the various sponsors can be hospitals, groups of physicians, insurance companies, unions, employers, and communities. Participants have access without further payment to all medical services around the clock, including preventive medical care. Unlike medical insurance plans, HMOs attempt to shift emphasis toward frequent and routine medical examination and the *prevention* of illness.

Experience with HMOs in practice has revealed some positive and negative developments. On the positive side, costs tend to be lower in HMOs. Hospitalization and the use of costly procedures go down, and preventive medicine is practiced more carefully. On the negative side, HMOs tend to curtail personnel and services in order to keep annual fees down. Surgery, for example, is delayed whenever possible. Furthermore, the plan subscriber has no choice in selecting a hospital and may be limited in choosing a doctor. Also, this plan provides no care for people who are unable to afford the annual fees of an HMO. If the goal of reform, therefore, is to extend adequate medical care to the poor, then HMOs are not a sufficient answer. There are those who say that the quality of care in HMOs is inferior, in part because the patient usually does not see the same physician on repeat visits. The Health Maintenance Act passed by the U.S. Congress in 1973 gave some impetus to the development of HMOs, but there still is significant resistance to their establishment in some areas of the country.

National health plans have been established in most industrialized countries. These plans are similar in some ways to HMOs, having similar advantages and disadvantages. They are, of course, not voluntary, for no citizen is excluded from these plans. In Britain, for example, the National Health Service seems to provide standard care at low cost to patients, but critics point out that there also seems to be a long waiting list for some nonstandard medical services. Patients frequently complain of a lack of continuity from visit to visit. Also, because the rate of escalating costs is approximately the same for countries with and without health service plans, this alternative does not significantly keep health costs down.

In the United States there have been some proposals for national health care service plans, but in reality they appear to have little chance of enactment. By contrast, proposals for national health *insurance* have waxed and waned in their likelihood of passage. Four kinds of schemes have been proposed:

1. granting tax credits to stimulate voluntary purchase of insurance from private companies;
2. extending Medicare and similar existing programs;
3. creating a national insurance agency similar to Social Security;
4. and requiring that insurance companies extend the opportunity for coverage to groups not now eligible—such as the self-employed, the poor, the elderly, and others.

The goal of each of these plans is to extend insurance coverage to all Americans, and each would reinforce the FFS model now in effect between doctor and patient. It is not surprising that critics see little hope that any one of these programs would correct the unequal distribution of limited health care resources, providing equal access to all citizens.

THE GOVERNMENT'S ROLE IN DISTRIBUTIVE JUSTICE

Underlying the debate discussed thus far is a concept we mentioned earlier—the concept of "distributive justice." The question is: What, if anything, do governments owe citizens? What do citizens have a *right* to expect their governments to do about making health care available? Did the woman whose bill was over $300,000 have a right to have that bill paid for by a hospital? the government? an insurance company? We must be careful here to avoid simplistic generalizations, but it is necessary to point out the underlying ethical assumptions in the argument. An examination of our assumptions helps us to understand why we hold the opinions we do, which brings us into the realm described in chapter 1 as *moral justification.*

The FFS model usually rests on a theory of distributive justice that has been called "free enterprise." It also has been said to rest on the "libertarian" theory of justice. Those who favor this system believe that the individual and his or her rights are paramount. The libertarian sees the physician as someone who, by hard work, has earned the right to offer medical services. For them, this is a right that should not be violated by society's priorities for the distribution of health care resources. Similarly, the right of the patient to seek whatever care he or she wants, and can afford, is an inviolate right. It follows naturally for the libertarian that because abilities, opportunities, and wealth are distributed unevenly in this society, access to health care too will be unevenly distributed. Any plan to *re*distribute health care resources more equitably is not an excuse for violating the rights of physicians and patients to enter into private FFS agreements. The libertarian would thus *not* permit a system in which a $300,000 bill is picked up by society, but an insurance system of voluntary plans and voluntary payments would be eminently acceptable.

In a sense, all plans other than FFS amount to attempts to redistribute health care resources. The motive may be a general ideal of equality or fairness, which is seen to be violated by factors of income, age, geographic location, or social status. Defenders of the FFS point out that health care has been provided to the poor through the Robin Hood system of setting fees (one using a sliding scale relating to ability to pay). Opponents point out that the Robin Hood system is arbitrary, irrational, and relies too much on the charity of individuals and institutions.

Behind most plans to modify or replace the libertarian (FFS) approach is one of two other theories of *distributive justice:* "egalitarian" theories and "utilitarian" theories. The egalitarian concept is rooted in deontological moral justifications, the utilitarian concept in the ethical theory by the same name. The egalitarian concept of distributive justice begins, as does the libertarian, with emphasis on the status and claims of individual persons. *This egalitarian deontological position deduces that all human beings are entitled to equal access to health care resources.* One defender of this theory, Charles Fried, has proposed that all citizens are entitled to a "decent *minimum* of health care." That is, each of us has a claim to, and society has an obligation to provide, a certain level of health care, which should be available to everyone, regardless of circumstances. The level recommended by Fried is a kind of baseline, below which no citizen should be allowed to fall. The $300,000 bill we have discussed would almost certainly *not* be picked up in full in his scheme.

Beyond the decent minimum, Fried would allow differences based on wealth, education, social status, and so on. After all, says Fried, medicine ought not to be subjected to a redistribution that is more radical than we apply to society's other benefits. Obviously this scheme would permit persons the liberty to spend $300,000 on a drug if they themselves picked up the cost. Another writer, John Rawls, favors a deontological egalitarian position that requires that all members of society receive the *maximum* level of society's benefits that *can* be shared on an equal basis—though here too there must be sharp limits to the costs. Rawls did not apply his theory to health care, but those who do would call for equal sharing of available health care resources. The point is that in the Rawlsian scheme of things such sharing is in general *morally required.*

The *utilitarian* concept of distributive justice is rooted in utilitarian ethical theory. (You might want to refer back to the theoretical discussion in chapter 1.) Consistent with utilitarian positions on other moral issues, this concept argues that we ought to allocate limited health care resources according to the principle of providing *the greatest good for the greatest number of people.* We should distribute health care in order to achieve low infant mortality rates throughout the population, a high longevity average, and so forth. The focus always is on the *aggregate* health of the *total* population. As you may suspect, utilitarians favor preventive medicine, the use of cost/benefit analysis, and public health programs over acute-care medicine. It is not likely in a utilitarian system that $300,000 would be made available for the treatment of one person, but the decision clearly is entirely a function of available resources in a utilitarian system, not a matter of claiming a "moral right."

There are significant criticisms in each of these three concepts of distributive justice. Many criticisms are, of course, linked to the deontological and utilitarian moral claims by which they have been justified. The FFS (libertarian) concept is based on a deontological justification that values maximizing an individual's freedom; it is concerned with redistributing health care for the benefit of the poor and those who live in remote locations only through charity. The *egalitarian* concept, also based on deontological moral claims (but reaching a very different conclusion), deals with the problem of unequal access. However, critics challenge its plausibility. It is too idealistic, they say; isn't it possible that for a period of time we will damage the health of the affluent, who have great potential contributions to make in society, while at the same time improving the health care of those people who have contributed least? The *utilitarian* concept of distributive justice in matters of health care faces the same objections that other utilitarian positions face in general. Utilitarians favor adequate health care for the statistical majority, but what about the fate of those individual persons outside the statistical majority? In its most extreme form, critics believe, strict utilitarian allocation of health care resources might lead us to withhold treatment from the young woman with the rare blood disease whose story began this chapter just because her expensive treatment would damage otherwise favorable statistics.

Each of the three points of view about health care distribution—libertarian, egalitarian, and utilitarian—has its strengths and weaknesses. Perhaps the only hope for a sufficient consensus lies in the debate over underlying moral assumptions. Perhaps you are beginning to feel that you can justify one of these positions more easily than others.

WHO SHOULD RECEIVE THE RESOURCES?

The problem of allocation of health care resources can be discussed in two stages. The first is *macroallocation,* which asks what portion of a society's wealth (for example, tax money) ought to go into which kinds of health care research or policies. Should public money be spent on a government campaign to decrease cigarette smoking in order to reduce the incidence of cancer and heart disease? Should public money be spent instead to find more sophisticated technologies for the treatment of cancer and heart disease? Once a treatment or technology has become available (for example, a totally implantable artificial heart), we face problems of *micro-allocation:* Who should receive that implantable heart, and who should not? Perhaps such hearts, which must be in short supply, should be allocated to males who are at the height of their earning power and their contributions to family and community. Is that acceptable?

Macroallocation decisions arise and are made one way or another by a society through its institutions—the Congress, the presidency, government agencies, private foundations—which embody political rhetoric and ideology, party platforms, and the causes of special interest groups. On the other hand, microallocation decisions arise and are made by individual health practitioners, boards of hospitals, insurance companies, and even individual patients and their families.

Microallocation choices often arise in situations similar to the following: Five patients suffering from kidney failure are awaiting a kidney transplant. A young accident victim's two kidneys become available. The usual tests are made, and it is determined that three of the five waiting patients are good matches for the available kidney. Conventional medical practice rules out the possibility of implanting the kidney in anyone for whom the prospect of a successful transplant is slim. Thus, there are three patients who seem to be equally qualified under present practice. How do we decide which two of the three will receive a kidney? This kind of situation has occurred with sufficient frequency to represent a real problem in modern medicine.

In actual practice, choices are made in three ways:

1. determining social merit, related to a judgment of the patient's ongoing contribution to family and society;

2. selecting on a first-come, first-served basis;
3. using some random lottery scheme (other than first-come, first-served).

Using *social worth* as a criterion is consistent with and usually derives from the utilitarian point of view. If society invests a valuable and perhaps scarce resource in one person over others, it therefore is entitled to consider the resulting good for the most people. In a sense, the individual health care practitioner becomes a "trustee" of society's interests. Those who disagree with the social-worth criterion say that a physician ought to concentrate all of his or her attention on the needs of the patient, without being distracted by concerns for society as a whole. Patients, for their part, need to feel reassured that the doctor is concerned primarily with their needs.

The random lottery approach to selecting recipients for scarce resources has not been used much in actual practice. Most frequently, the first-come, first-served approach is used. This practice tends to avoid the problems associated with utilitarian selection. Patients are treated more equitably, patients maintain faith in their doctors, and discrimination against "undesirable" persons is lessened. But, decision-making is left to luck.

DIFFICULT CHOICES

The decisions faced in microallocation and macroallocation are difficult. They can represent dilemmas of the most acute kind and must sometimes be made almost overnight. On the one hand, we see that the awesome developments of modern medicine give us the capacity to preserve lives that in an earlier time would have been surrendered to fate. On the other hand, the sophistication and cost of these measures make some of them extremely scarce. To date, especially in the United States, macroallocation choices have tended to favor more and more spending for further development of sophisticated medical technology, typically available only in large medical centers located in urban areas. Only recently has this tendency come into question, as skyrocketing costs claim an increasing chunk of our total resources. At the same time, there is growing pressure to achieve a more equitable distribution of health resources. We have gone from the era of virtually unlimited funding, research, and development in medicine to an era in which choices must be made about what to pursue and what *not* to pursue.

These are significant developments that cannot be abstracted from political theories of the proper role of the State; they represent a shift from a time and a perspective to which we probably cannot return. In the past, our societal view permitted the assumption of unlimited resources of many kinds. We felt that we could pursue many forms of development with equal intensity. Now we are becoming aware that many kinds of resources, including complex medical technology, must be treated as scarcities. If we cannot pursue all avenues that provide human services with equal intensity, then we must *choose*. If the previous era was one of "naive optimism," then perhaps the next should be referred to as an era of "difficult choices." These choices are, as we have attempted to demonstrate, moral choices which frequently lie just beneath the process of making public policy in a democratic society. Sometimes they emerge with startling clarity in the actual work of governmental agencies and commissions.

Perhaps this theoretical discourse will take on more significance if we provide another real example. Let us consider the development and distribution choices related to the so-called "artificial heart."

THE CASE OF THE TOTALLY IMPLANTABLE ARTIFICIAL HEART

The totally implantable artificial heart (TIAH), made of synthetic material, was designed for severely threatened cardiac patients as a replacement for heart function. The motor that drives it, and its power source, are totally and permanently implanted in the body of the recipient, so that it replaces the natural heart completely. Several experimental designs are under development, but no TIAH has come into use yet. By the time the artificial heart is perfected, millions of dollars will have been spent in research and development. The cost per patient probably will range between $25,000 and $75,000 each. In anticipation of the development of the TIAH, the National Lung and Heart Institute established a panel to deal with public policy questions of macroallocation and microallocation. The macroallocation questions under consideration were: Should this society, through its government, fund the costly development of a TIAH? Should a nuclear-powered model be developed, or should we concentrate on a battery-powered model instead? The microallocation question was: Should criteria be established to insure fair distribution of the TIAH once it is perfected and available on the market? The work of the panel and of subsequent writers have provided a record of how choices of distributive justice are confronted and how working conclusions were reached in this particular case.

The panel was succinct in dealing with the microallocation question. Their conclusion was:

In the event artificial heart resources are in scarce supply, decisions as to the selection of candidates for the implantation of the artificial heart should be made by physicians and medical institutions on the basis of medical criteria. If the pool of patients with medical needs exceed supply, procedures should be devised for some form of random selection. Social worth criteria should not be used, and every effort should be exerted to minimize the possibility that social worth may implicitly be taken into account.[5]

The panel also dealt with several questions of macroallocation, the first one being, "Should government funds be used for the development of a medical technology that would benefit only a relatively small part of the population, or should government funds be used for preventive medicine which might decrease the possibility for heart disease for many in the population?"[6] The choice between *preventive* and *rescue* medicine is a familiar one. Because cardiac disease is a leading cause of death in the United States, and considering that as many as 25,000 persons annually might benefit from the development of the TIAH, the panel saw no philosophical or public policy objections to the development of a mechanical heart.

The panel also considered the macroallocation question of whether to recommend development of a nuclear-powered or battery-powered TIAH. The nuclear-powered heart would be reliable, efficient, and longer-lived than the battery-powered heart, but the effects of prolonged exposure to low level radiation might be harmful to the heart recipient or others. Note that while the recipient in principle could choose to gamble with its long-term effects, we still would not know what possible damage might occur to others, including the unborn. The panel finally recommended development of *both* kinds of artificial hearts, but advised less actual experimental application of the nuclear-powered model, at least until side effects could be better documented and understood.

The recommendations of this panel—indeed its very existence—point to a new era in health care and public policy. Long-range decision-making, especially with thorough consideration of the moral aspects of public policy, is still rare today. But, probably for the first time, a sincere effort was made to anticipate and plan for the eventual effects of new developments in medical technology.

We remind you that underlying all such deliberations and recommendations are concepts of distributive justice. In his summary of the work of the panel, one member, Albert Jonsen, wrote as follows: "Behind both difficult problems—availability and selection [of those who will receive a TIAH]—stands the thesis that every person has a 'right to health care.'

5. Albert R. Jonsen, "The Totally Implantable Artificial Heart," *Hastings Center Report* 3 (November 1973): 1–4.
6. Ibid.

Neither indigence nor social 'unworthiness' are sufficient reasons to bar a person from health care needed to sustain health and life."[7]

Other commentators have written about the issues that faced the panel. Predictably, their points of view tend to fragment along lines of the particular form of libertarian, egalitarian, or utilitarian theory that they accept as a correct approach to distributive justice. A libertarian argues that the physician/medical researcher must have the freedom to pursue whatever development he or she deems worthy, and, moreover, when the TIAH is ready for use, the available hearts should go to those recipients who *can pay* for the hearts and who *wish to* do so. Their "liberties" too must not be constrained by a federal system of allocation. In other words, allocation should proceed on a free-market basis, with everyone's rights of noninterference protected.

Egalitarians for the most part argue for each citizen's right to some decent *minimum* of health care that will in principle be distributed without encumbrance to all in the society who *need* it. Egalitarians might not, however, push for the development of the TIAH as a government-funded project and also need not seek to prohibit its manufacture and purchase by those who could afford it. The egalitarian notion of a "decent minimum" would be exceeded by such an expensive and limited item. Thus, assuming that insurance carriers refused to cover the total cost of the TIAH, only those who could supplement the cost out of personal income would receive the hearts. But what about those egalitarians of whom there are a few, who argue for an equal *maximum* level of health care for all citizens? Probably they would argue for investment of public health funds in preventive medicine in preference to the development of a sophisticated and costly device such as the TIAH. They might then reconsider the question if all citizens at some point reach an equal, high level of basic health.

Utilitarians would want to maximize the total good, versus the losses, for the largest number of people. For example, they clearly would favor the TIAH (and its public funding) if it could be demonstrated that the device would decrease morbidity and mortality due to heart disease in the *total* population and would be cost-effective in the economy. Again, they might favor the heart if they believed it would reduce the society's costs in caring for people with heart disease. They might want to extend some other form of health care compensation—for example, increased insurance coverage at a commensurate amount to cover other afflictions—to those members of society who stand to gain very little personally from the development of the TIAH.

7. Ibid.

Imagine you are a member of a national panel assigned to make macroallocation and microallocation decisions regarding the development and distribution of a significant, new medical technology like the TIAH.

1. Would you vote for a new technology that tended to make a significant contribution to preventive medicine over one promoting rescue medicine?
2. Would you vote for or against the use of federal money to fund the research and development of such a technology, with specific guidelines for the researchers engaged? Or, should the federal government stay out of such activities and leave research and development to universities, businesses, or perhaps a private foundation, such as the American Heart Association?
3. What criteria would you endorse for distribution of the new technology?
   a. No regulations at all. Let those who can afford it make use of it.
   b. Generally, let those who can afford it, or have adequate insurance, or are covered by an existing federal program, make use of it—with some effort to make it available to others whose continued life would be valuable to the society.
   c. Establish a strict system of equal distribution of a first-come, first-served basis, with no regard for social worth or ability to pay.
4. Of the three concepts of distributive justice discussed—libertarian, egalitarian and utilitarian—with which *one* are your answers most consistent? Did any of your answers surprise you?

WORKING OUR WAY FROM THEORY TO PRACTICE

It is virtually impossible to adopt a position and discuss proposed courses of action in matters like these without appealing to the underlying assumptions. Superficial discussion at the public policy level seldom leads to satisfying public policy decisions. The implementation of a government program or policy is the end result of a chain of moral reasoning and almost always based on accepted legal rights, dignified by the courts. In turn, the argumentation and deliberation of the courts, which establishes legal rights, inevitably must refer back to claims of more encompassing moral rights. These claimed moral rights are best understood in terms of their underlying concepts of distributive justice. Finally, underlying various concepts of distributive justice are the various forms of deontological and utilitarian ethical theory. What this means is that if you, and we as a society, wish to work toward deep understanding and consensus as a basis for our policies, then we must weigh alternatives that reach all the way back to our most basic ethical assumptions of distributive justice. The diagram below may help you to visualize a chain of steps linking broad theory to specific policy.

An ethical theory (deontological or utilitarian)
↓
Concepts of distributive justice
↓
Claims of moral rights
↓
Establishment of legal rights
↓
Implementation of programs and policies to govern behavior

The issues and examples discussed in this chapter are the tip of a vast iceberg of issues that will emerge during the remaining few years of the twentieth century. In the sense that we do not yet have answers ready for these issues, then we are *not ready for modern medicine.* We have *not* decided how much health care and modern medical technology should go around, nor to whom it should go. In an atmosphere of increasingly scarce resources, we have *not* found a satisfying balance between expenditures for preventive medicine and expenditures for treatment. We are discovering that we do not have the resources any longer to do everything that could be done in health care. Among the vast repertoire of medical procedures which we *can* perform, we have *not* been able to draw a consistent distinction between those which *ought* to be carried out and those which should *not.*

Issues of allocation are at the heart of all disciplines related to economic and social theory, and they have been with us since the beginnings of human society. Now, in a world of exponentially increasing social and technical complexity, models of distributive justice form a fulcrum on which we must balance policies of modern medicine. Our personal and societal expectations of health and life and death sway to and fro in the balance. The choices we make will reflect our values, the sort of society we are, and the kind of society we want to become.

SELECTED READINGS
There Is No Right to Health Care . . .[8]

The current debate on health care in the United States is of the first order of importance to the health professions, and of no less importance to the political

8. Excerpts from Robert M. Sade, "Medical Care as a Right: A Refutation," excerpted by permission of the *New England Journal of Medicine* 285 (1971): 1288 ff.

future of the nation, for precedents are now being set that will be applied to the rest of American society in the future. In the enormous volume of verbiage that has poured forth, certain fundamental issues have been so often misrepresented that they have now become commonly accepted fallacies. This paper will be concerned with the most important of these misconceptions, that health care is a right, as well as a brief consideration of some of its corollary fallacies.

The concept of rights has its roots in the moral nature of man and its practical expression in the political system that he creates. Both morality and politics must be discussed before the relation between political rights and health care can be appreciated.

A "right" defines a freedom of action. For instance, a right to a material object is the uncoerced choice of the use to which that object will be put; a right to a specific action, such as free speech, is the freedom to engage in that activity without forceful repression. The moral foundation of the rights of man begins with the fact that he is a living creature: he has the right to his own life. All other rights are corollaries of this primary one; without the right to life, there can be no others, and the concept of rights itself becomes meaningless.

The freedom to live, however, does not automatically ensure life. For man, a specific course of action is required to sustain his life, a course of action that must be guided by reason and reality and has as its goal the creation or acquisition of material values, such as food and clothing, and intellectual values, such as self-esteem and integrity. His moral system is the means by which he is able to select the values that will support his life and achieve his happiness. . . .

The concept of medical care as the patient's right is immoral because it denies the most fundamental of all rights, that of a man to his own life and the freedom of action to support it. Medical care is neither a right nor a privilege: it is a service that is provided by doctors and others to people who wish to purchase it. It is the provision of this service that a doctor depends upon for his livelihood, and is his means of supporting his own life. If the right to health care belongs to the patient, he starts out owning the services of a doctor without the necessity of either earning them or receiving them as a gift from the only man who has the right to give them: the doctor himself. . . . American medicine is now at the point in the story where the state has proclaimed the nonexistent "right" to medical care as a fact of public policy, and has begun to pass the laws to enforce it. The doctor finds himself less and less his own master and more and more controlled by forces outside of his own judgment. . . .

The basic fallacy that health care is a right has led to several corollary fallacies, among them the following:

That health is primarily a community or social rather than an individual concern.[a] A simple calculation from American mortality statistics[b] quickly corrects that false concept: 67 per cent of deaths in 1967 were due to diseases known

a. J. S. Millis, "Wisdom? Health? Can Society Guarantee Them?" *New England Journal of Medicine* 283 (1970): 260–61.

b. H. Shoeck, ed., *Financing Medical Care: An Appraisal of Foreign Programs* (Caldwell, Idaho: Caxton Printers, 1962); M. J. Lynch and S. S. Raphael, *Medicine and the State* (Springfield, Ill.: Charles C. Thomas, 1963).

to be caused or exacerbated by alcohol, tobacco smoking or overeating, or were due to accidents. Each of those factors is either largely or wholly correctable by individual action. Although no statistics are available, it is likely that morbidity, with the exception of common respiratory infections, has a relation like that of mortality to personal habits and excesses.

That state medicine has worked better in other countries than free enterprise has worked here. There is no evidence to support that contention, other than anecdotal testimonals and the spurious citation of infant mortality and longevity statistics. There is, on the other hand, a good deal of evidence to the contrary.

That the provision of medical care somehow lies outside the laws of supply and demand, and that government-controlled health care will be free care. In fact, no service or commodity lies outside the economic laws. Regarding health care, market demand, individual want, and medical need are entirely different things, and have a very complex relation with the cost and the total supply of available care, as recently discussed and clarified by Jeffers et al.[c] They point out that " 'health is purchaseable,' meaning that somebody has to pay for it, individually or collectively, at the expense of foregoing the current or future consumption of other things." The question is whether the decision of how to allocate the consumer's dollar should belong to the consumer or to the state. It has already been shown that the choice of how a doctor's services should be rendered belongs only to the doctor: in the same way the choice of whether to buy a doctor's service rather than some other commodity or service belongs to the consumer as a logical consequence of the right to his own life.

That opposition to national health legislation is tantamount to opposition to progress in health care. Progress is made by the free interaction of free minds developing new ideas in an atmosphere conducive to experimentation and trial. If group practice really is better than solo, we will find out because the success of groups will result in more groups (which has, in fact, been happening); if prepaid comprehensive care really is the best form of practice, it will succeed and the health industry will swell with new Kaiser–Permanente plans. But let one of these or any other form of practice become the law, and the system is in a straitjacket that will stifle progress. Progress requires freedom of action, and that is precisely what national health legislation aims at restricting.

That doctors should help design the legislation for a national health system, since they must live with and within whatever legislation is enacted. To accept this concept is to concede to the opposition its philosophic premises, and thus to lose the battle. The means by which nonproducers and hangers-on throughout history have been able to expropriate material and intellectual values from the producers has been identified only relatively recently: the sanction of the victim.[d] Historically, few people have lost their freedom and their rights without some degree of complexity in the plunder. If the American medical profession accepts the concept of health care as the right of the patient, it will have earned the

c. J. R. Jeffers, M. F. Bognanno, and J. C. Bartlett, "On the Demand versus Need for Medical Services and the Concept of 'Shortage,' " *American Journal of Public Health* 61 (1971): 46–63.

d. A. Rand, *Atlas Shrugged* (New York: Random House, 1957), p. 1066.

Kennedy–Griffiths bill by default. The alternative for any health professional is to withhold his sanction and make clear who is being victimized. Any physician can say to those who would shackle his judgment and control his profession: I do not recognize your right to my life and my mind, which belong to me and me alone; I will not participate in any legislated solution to any health problem.

In the face of the raw power that lies behind government programs, nonparticipation is the only way in which personal values can be maintained. And it is only with the attainment of the highest of those values—integrity, honesty and self-esteem—that the physician can achieve his most important professional value, the absolute priority of the welfare of his patients.

The preceding discussion should not be interpreted as proposing that there are no problems in the delivery of medical care. Problems such as high cost, few doctors, low quantity of available care in economically depressed area may be real, but it is naïve to believe that governmental solutions through coercive legislation can be anything but shortsighted and formulated on the basis of political expediency. The only long-range plan that can hope to provide for the day after tomorrow is a "nonsystem"—that is, a system that proscribes the imposition by force (legislation) of any one group's conception of the best forms of medical care. We must identify our problems and seek to solve them by experimentation and trial in an atmosphere of freedom from compulsion. Our sanction of anything less will mean the loss of our personal values, the death of our profession, and a heavy blow to political liberty.

. . . But Perhaps There Ought to Be a Right to Health Care[9]

Should the goods and services required to preserve and restore our health be bought and sold in the marketplace, like television sets and haircuts, or should they be provided in some other way? To give a complete answer to this question we would have to take into account a wide variety of considerations. We would need to inquire into the economics of alternative schemes for providing health care. We could not reach a proper decision unless we knew whether one scheme provided health care at a significantly lower cost than another. We would also need information of a sociological nature: who would receive care under the different schemes, and what kind of care? Even after we had all the economic and sociological information that we would reasonably expect to acquire, however, some very fundamental questions would remain. These would be ethical questions. What are our ends or values? What is it that we are trying to achieve in this area? What are the values or principles that should guide our choice between alternative methods of distribution? What is our conception of a good society, and how does this conception affect our choice of method?

It is these ethical questions that I am going to explore in this chapter. They cannot be considered in isolation from economic and sociological issues, and so I shall be referring to these areas in the course of the chapter, but my focus will be ethical. . . .

9. Excerpts from Peter Singer, "Freedoms and Utilities in the Distribution of Health Care," in *Ethics and Public Policy*, ed. Robert Veatch and Roy Branson, pp. 175–92. Reprinted with permission from *Ethics and Health Policy*, copyright 1976, Ballinger Publishing Co.

Health Care as a Right   It is very common nowadays for those dissatisfied with
the market approach to the distribution of health care to claim that "health care is
a right." Thus Senator Abraham Ribicoff, a leading campaigner for health reform
in this country and chairman of a Senate subcommittee that has investigated
aspects of medical care, argues in his new book that the most basic need is for "a
new way of thinking about medical care, a philosophy that states our belief that to
receive medical care is the individual's right, but to provide it is the nation's
privilege."[a]

It should not be difficult to find other expressions of the idea that health care is a
right. The phrase has a forceful ring to it, and it makes a fine slogan. If we
interpret the slogan as saying that everyone should have a legal right to obtain
health care free of charge, we have no problem in understanding the claim,
although of course it needs argument to back it up; but if we try to take the idea
that "health care is a right" literally, as if this idea in itself is all the justification
needed for making health care a legal right, we will find it difficult to know what
to make of this claim.

How are we to establish that health care really is a right? Argument soon comes
to a halt. It is impossible to get people to agree on any list of natural or human
rights, once we get beyond the right to life, and even that is rarely held to be
absolute. Other rights, like the right to vote, depend on a particular political
context. So-called "welfare rights," of which the right to health care would be one,
are more puzzling still, since they require not merely that others leave me alone or
refrain from doing something to me, but also that others take some positive action
to provide me with something. So while we can, in almost any circumstances,
claim that to kill someone without his consent is to violate his right to life, we can
only speak meaningfully of a violation of a right to health care if a society has
reached the level of sophistication at which it has the means and knowledge to
provide health care for everyone. The fact that the possibility of talking of a "right
to health care" depends on available resources suggests, however, that it is a right
that must be balanced against other possible uses of those resources—and this
suggests that whether we finally do decide to recognize a right to health care will
depend on a complex assessment of the benefits of providing free health care, as
compared with the benefits of alternative systems of health care distribution. . . .

Distributive Justice   A second claim that has seemed to some to settle the problem of whether health care should be taken out of the marketplace is the idea that
it is obviously unjust to provide health care on any other grounds than those of
need. Justice, it is commonly and I think correctly said, demands that we treat like
cases alike, except when there is a relevant difference between them. In the case of
the distribution of health care, is it not self-evident that the only relevant consideration is how great a person's need for care is? Money, how wealthy a person is,
obviously has nothing at all to do with whether he should receive medical
care. . . .

. . . Personally, I think this really is an ideal form of distribution, if it can be

a. Abraham Ribicoff, *The American Medical Machine* (New York: Harrow Books, 1972), p. 10.

made to work, but the fact that it is a quite general principle means that it cannot be invoked by those who claim that health care is *specially* unsuited to the marketplace. . . .

Freedom   The marketplace is most often defended as a method of distributing goods and services, including health care, by those who see themselves as defenders of freedom. . . . The case of health care allows us to examine the assumption that leaving distribution to the market does increase freedom. . . .

In an open market the individual doctor would be less secure, economically, than he is at present. Economic considerations would therefore, become more prominent in the doctor's relationship with his patient. The patient would be aware of this, and might come to suspect self-interested considerations when the doctor advises frequent visits or further treatment. So market considerations could undermine the relationship between the doctor and his patient. The A.M.A. places a great deal of emphasis on this relationship, and I believe it is right to do so. Medical practice would be changed for the worse if a patient could not trust his doctor, confident that the doctor's motivation was exclusively a concern for his patient's well-being. . . .

A National Health Service?   A national health service must be financed by taxation. It does, therefore, limit the freedom of the taxpayer to decide for himself how much he shall spend on health, and how much on other items. Of course, other welfare measures like social security do the same, in their own area. There is, however, a prima facie case against such a restriction. What can be said in defense of the restriction in this case?

First, it may be that the community, acting together, can achieve goods that the individual could not achieve, no matter how much he decided to spend on health care. We have already seen examples of this in respect of obtaining cheap, uncontaminated blood and obtaining medical services that have not been distorted by the threat of malpractice suits. There are many other ways in which the special nature of medical care may make it unsuited to market control. For instance, the market's answer to the uncertainty of an individual's need for extensive medical care is private insurance. Private insurance, however, tends to be extremely expensive for ordinary visits to a doctor, because a doctor, in the privacy of his office, is not subject to supervision from his peers or anyone else, and so might prescribe unnecessary treatment in order to increase his remuneration from the insurance company. One consequence of this is that most people are insured for hospital visits, but not for office visits; and a consequence of this is that some medical care now takes place in hospitals that would be done more economically in the patient's home or the doctor's office. The ultimate consequence is that the consumer pays more for his medical insurance.

This difficulty is not one that can be eliminated simply by a system of national health insurance like those envisaged in recent congressional bills. These proposals would retain the principle of paying the doctor for each treatment, and this would leave the system wide open to abuse if it covered office visits, unless there were a huge and expensive system of inspectors. On the other hand, if the scheme does not cover office visits, it will accelerate the trend to increased hospitalization.

This problem can be avoided under a national health service, by paying the doctor on some basis other than the cost of the treatment he prescribes. In Britain, for example, doctors are paid according to the number of patients on their roll, with a lower payment per patient after a certain figure is reached to discourage excessively large rolls, and an absolute ceiling at a higher point, to prohibit unworkably large practices. Admittedly there are drawbacks to this method too, for a doctor gets paid even if he does very little for his patients. A complaints procedure and the possibility of patients transferring to another doctor may curb this tendency. A more important restraint is the bond of an ethical relationship between doctor and patient that has not been eroded by the commercialization of medical practice. . . .

The final justification for overriding the freedom of each to spend his income as he prefers is one that relates to a theme that has run through this chapter: the nature of the community that we live in. Here we must consider whether it is not desirable that a community be integrated in certain fundamental areas of life, rather than being divided along lines of class or race. As Brian Barry has noted, the promotion of this value distinguishes a national health service from a system of universal insurance that provides standard sums of money for given treatments, while leaving doctors and hospitals to charge what they will, and the patient to make up the difference if he selects a doctor or hospital that charges above the standard amount. This insurance system would provide a basic level of care for everyone.[b] I do not agree with Barry that this value is the *only* one that distinguishes these two systems of providing health care (I have suggested others in this chapter); but it is true that universal insurance would provide many of the benefits of a national health service, including redistribution and the provision of security for all against the threat of ruinous expenditure on medical care. What the insurance proposal could not do, however, is provide an integrated health service that is used by people of all classes and races. We would still have one standard of care for the wealthy and another for the poor.

How important is integration in the area of medicine? It does not seem to be as important as in education, for it does not determine a person's opportunities for the whole of his life to the extent that education does (although medicine may do this in exceptional cases). Still, there are important reasons for desiring integration in medicine too. As Barry says, "so long as those with money can buy exemption from the common lot the rulers and the generally dominant groups in a society will have little motive for making sure that the public facilities are of good quality." In other words, if we want good public facilities, we have to ensure that those who can complain effectively when standards are allowed to drop use the facilities.

A more fundamental aspect of integration is that it makes a substantial difference to the image that we have of our community. The knowledge that when it

b. Brian Barry, *Political Argument* (New York: The Humanities Press, 1965), chap. 7.

comes to vital things like medical care we are all in it together, and your money cannot buy you anything that I am not equally entitled to, may do a good deal to mitigate the effects of inequality in other less vital areas, and create the atmosphere of community concern for all that I have already discussed.

This last consideration is the first one we have encountered that goes beyond even what the British National Health Service has achieved. Private medicine does exist in Britain, and very wealthy people do sometimes get treatment that the National Health Service does not provide. Money may allow one to go down to London and be operated on by an outstanding surgeon, while a person who could not afford this would have to accept the general level of surgery in the area in which he lived. Yet this is not a major problem. Because of the generally high standard of treatment that the National Health Service provides at no cost, and the high costs of private medicine, only a very few people avail themselves of private treatment. Of those who do, by no means all actually do receive treatment that is superior to that offered by the National Health Service. So long as private medicine remains such a minor part of health care as a whole, it does not seem necessary to take the step of prohibiting it altogether. Allowing private medicine to exist, can, as Barry suggests, be seen as a reasonable compromise between the values of freedom and integration.

ANNOTATED BIBLIOGRAPHY
Books and Articles

Beauchamp, Tom L., and James F. Childress. *Princples of Biomedical Ethics.* New York: Oxford University Press, 1979. Chap. 6. An approach to many problems of access and allocation through moral principles of justice and their application.

Fein, Rashi. "On Achieving Access and Equity in Health Care." *Milbank Memorial Fund Quarterly* 50 (October 1972): 157–90. An economist writes about fair access to health care.

Havighurst, Clark C. "The Ethics of Cost Control in Medical Care." *Soundings* 60 (Spring 1977): 22–39. A lawyer writes about the importance of an analytical approach to cost control.

Katz, Jay, and Alexander M. Capron. *Catastrophic Diseases: Who Decides What? A Psychological and Legal Analysis.* New York: Russell Sage Foundation, 1975. A careful and detailed volume on the nature of decisions about funding treatment for catastrophic diseases and about the proper treatment of patients.

Anthologies

Beauchamp, Tom L., and LeRoy Walters, eds. *Contemporary Issues in Bioethics.* 2nd ed. Belmont, Calif.: Wadsworth Publishing Company, Inc., 1982. Chaps. 9, 10. Contains many basic articles on the subjects addressed in this chapter.

Shelp, Earl, ed. *Justice and Health Care.* Boston: D. Reidel, 1981. A very well-constructed volume on justice and access to health care. It is predominantly philosophical in approach.

Veatch, Robert M., and Roy Branson, eds. *Ethics and Health Policy*. Cambridge, Mass.: Ballinger Publishing Co., 1975. This influential, widely quoted volume contains several extremely important essays, perhaps most prominently those by Robert Veatch and Peter Singer.

Articles from the *Encyclopedia of Bioethics*

Health Care
  I. Health-Care System *Philip R. Lee and Carol Emmott*
  II. Humanization and Dehumanization of Health Care *Jan Howard*
  III. Right to Health-Care Services *Albert R. Jonsen*
  IV. Theories of Justice and Health Care *Roy Branson*
Health as an Obligation *Samuel Gorovitz*
Health Insurance *Stefan A. Riesenfeld*
Health Policy
  I. Evolution of Health Policy *Stephen P. Strickland*
  II. Health Policy in International Perspective *Odin W. Anderson*

Literature

Chekhov, Anton. "Gusev." In *The Portable Chekhov*, ed. Ayrahm Yarmolinsky. New York: Viking Press, 1965. Chekhov, another doctor-writer, was by far the most prolific, writing some 800 short stories. In this story, the treatment (or more accurately, the mistreatment) of poor patients is explored: "You don't pay them [doctors] any money, you are a nuisance, and you spoil their statistics with your deaths." Although most people assume modern medicine treats poor patients better than those described by Chekhov, this story still raises the question of how a society and its health care practitioners treat those at the bottom of the economic ladder.

Audio/Visual

"The Malady of Health Care." "NOVA" series, 55-minute film or videotape. Sale or rental, Time/Life Video, Eisenhower Drive, Paramus, N.J. 07652. This episode surveys the three modes of health care discussed in this chapter—fee-for-service, health maintenance organizations, and national health service—by examining their actual performance in the U.S. and the United Kingdom.

8

APPLIED GENETICS—INFORMATION
AND INTERVENTION

Once it is alive as a separate entity on the face of this planet, each organism tends to behave or adapt in ways that will preserve or extend its own life. Goldfish and goldenrod and gold-traders tend to seek nourishment and protection from predators and harmful extremes in environment each day and night. Furthermore, each species adapts physically, biologically over thousands of years in ways that allow its members to survive more easily. This adaptive effect is cumulative upon the species, so that each new member of that species carries into its life a legacy from past lives.

Humankind has developed a highly refined nervous system, and with it the power to wonder, to search for the regularities of the universe and reflect upon them, to rationalize in abstract terms, and to think about ourselves. No other species of life even approaches *Homo sapiens* in this respect. Inevitably, we have wondered about the amazing mechanism by which each new organism, including ourselves, inherits its structure and biology. We invented the science of genetics as a means of finding answers to these questions. Over a century ago the Augustinian monk, Gregor Mendel, documented the probabilities of inheritance, and in the late 1950s James Watson and Francis Crick discovered the structure of the DNA (deoxyribonucleic acid) molecule responsible for carrying biological information from one generation to the next.

What has happened is unprecedented in the entire history of life: we have discovered the templates, the blueprints, of life, including our own, and we are learning to read them, to redraw them, and apply them in biological and medical research.

GENETICS AND EUGENICS

Common-sense observation reveals that offspring inherit the characteristics of their parents. Farmers knew this for centuries and used the knowledge to breed animals that would be stronger or more productive, or yield more meat or resist disease.

But it was Mendel, closely observing and recording successive generations of garden peas, who deduced that there are dominant traits and recessive traits and who speculated on the existence of a physical mechanism controlling genetic transmission. Although he published his observations in the 1860s, it was not until after 1900 that his work was rediscovered and linked with a flurry of activity by geneticists who were rapidly closing in on the function of "inherited particles," or *genes*, as they were labeled.

Also in the nineteenth century, a cousin of Charles Darwin, Sir Frances Galton, introduced another important idea: if through selective breeding superior breeds of farm animals can be produced, it ought to be just as easy "to produce a highly gifted race of men." He called his idea *eugenics*. Although the idea of matching men and women to produce "superior" children was at least as old as Plato's *Republic*, the growing awareness of genetics and evolution brought attention to Galton's idea of superior breeding of human beings. *Negative eugenics* sought to discourage reproduction by people with "undesirable traits," and *positive eugenics* sought to encourage those with "desirable" traits to reproduce.

Negative eugenics was sometimes translated into public policy. In 1907 Indiana became the first state to enact a sterilization law. The legislation required nonvoluntary sterilization of confirmed criminals, idiots, and others in state institutions. By 1931 thirty states had passed sterilization laws. Similarly, immigration laws were designed to keep out "undesirable" nationalities. Underlying sterilization and immigration laws of the early twentieth century was a belief that the "purity" of the race must be protected—a tenet which, of course, produced unimaginable torture and death under Adolf Hitler.

Still, the idea persists that certain clear-cut criteria of desirable and undesirable human traits can be linked directly to genetic inheritance. Just a few years ago, the belief that an extra Y chromosome in certain males accounted for their criminal behavior actually produced some state laws and hospital policies to screen all male newborns to detect those with an extra Y chromosome. More recently, it has been observed that *many* males have an extra Y chromosome, most of whom exhibit no extraordinarily aggressive behavior, much less criminal behavior.

Subsequent developments in genetics have greatly increased our understanding of the mechanism of inheritance and methods of detecting genetic disorders, but have resulted in only a very limited capacity to correct or treat genetic disorders, so far. In the 1950s, Crick and Watson announced their ideas of the structure of DNA. Some writers have compared their breakthrough to the discovery of the atom. The fundamental shape of DNA explained how genes were strung out on long strands. Other scientists soon discovered how these genes formed a "language" which, through a series of chemical reactions, instructed the development of an organism. Genes were soon called the building blocks or the blueprints of life. Understand how genes work and you might understand how an organism, even as complex as a human being, develops its physiological traits. Through laboratory analysis, geneticists might "read" the genetic "language" and know, for example, whether an adult is an unwitting carrier of a genetic disorder or whether a fetus or a newborn is affected by a genetic disorder whose symptoms will not manifest themselves for months or even years after birth. By analyzing the genetic material in a blood or tissue cell from an adult or a newborn, through what is now known as *genetic testing,* such questions might one day be answered. By the late 1960s a new kind of genetic testing had been introduced, amniocentesis, which we discussed in chapter 2.

By the early 1970s, some states required genetic testing on a mass basis. The first genetic disorder for which most states enacted routine screening of newborns was a disorder called PKU, short for phenylketonuria. It had been discovered that if infants with PKU were put on a restrictive diet immediately the debilitating aspects of the disease could be offset. For those who were discovered through mandatory genetic screening to have PKU, a successful therapy was available, but for many other genetic diseases there were and still are no successful therapies.

GENETIC ENGINEERING

In 1973 there came about another significant development whose ramifications we are still trying to understand fully. Once the structure of DNA had been discovered and its "language" deciphered, the next step was to manipulate genetic material itself. Called formally *DNA recombination* and informally "genetic engineering" or "gene splicing," these procedures involve actually cutting and rearranging genetic material. The result is that the subsequent development of the organism can be altered.

There are many possible benefits from genetic engineering. If genetic disorders can be detected, then perhaps through genetic engineering they can be corrected.

Producing rare body chemicals in quantity through recombinant DNA technologies is promising, too. For example, it might be possible to make plentiful, inexpensive insulin for diabetics. Hormones, produced by recombinant DNA technologies, could be administered to dwarves early in life to bring about more nearly normal growth. Interferon, a protein substance in the body that appears to inhibit infection, is being studied for its possible value in combatting multiple sclerosis and cancer. Medical researchers are seeking to produce interferon in quantity through genetic engineering.

Still, reservations have been raised. The exotic and unknown nature of DNA research caused a moratorium in the 1970s. That has been lifted, and once stringent federal guidelines have been relaxed. The conceivable use of genetic engineering for warfare has raised some concern. *Cloning* is another genetic engineering feat that has received widespread attention. The nucleus of a reproductive cell is replaced with the nucleus of another cell, so that the resulting new organism replicates the characteristics of the introduced nucleus. The new organism does not receive half its genes from each parent, as in normal reproduction, but duplicates the genetic make-up of parent. Cloning has been accomplished in laboratory mice, but not in human beings—yet. The largest of all questions raised by developments in genetics is the question of *purpose*. What *ought* to be the *purpose* of the application of new and developing knowledge and technologies in genetics?

Through genetic testing of adults who want to be parents, we can detect carriers of genetic diseases and know the odds of their producing children who will be affected. A straightforward application of Mendel's laws of heredity produces the following odds: If both parents are carriers of a genetic disorder, the odds are fifty percent of their having a child who is a *carrier,* twenty-five percent for a child who is *affected,* and twenty-five percent for a *normal* child. If one parent is affected and the other is neither affected nor a carrier, any child born has a fifty percent chance of being *affected* and a fifty percent chance of *neither being affected nor a carrier.* These chances do not hold for each child conceived because there are, of course, exceptions when these chances do not hold up strictly.

By testing adults and newborns, specialists can detect individuals who have inherited some genetic diseases, even though no symptoms have yet presented themselves. Through amniocentesis and other prenatal genetic testing technologies, it is possible to identify fetuses that will be affected by genetic disorders or will be carriers. Right now, through selective abortion, such fetuses can be destroyed. In the future, successful treatments and even cures may be found. All indications are that future strides in genetic engineering will bring us closer to successful therapy. For now, however, in most cases we can *detect* but not *treat* effectively. Future developments in genetic engineering may provide not only the capacity for gene therapy, but also opportunities to *design* future generations.

What effect will all this have on the evolution of the species? This question requires scientific and political attention now, and answers will not come easily. Already, through an intensive, routine genetic prenatal

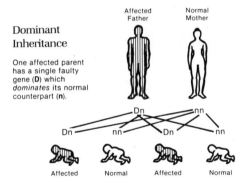

Dominant Inheritance

One affected parent has a single faulty gene (**D**) which *dominates* its normal counterpart (**n**).

Chances of inheriting either the **D** or the **n** from the affected parent are 50%, for *each* child.

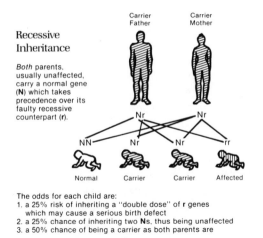

Recessive Inheritance

Both parents, usually unaffected, carry a normal gene (**N**) which takes precedence over its faulty recessive counterpart (**r**).

The odds for each child are:
1. a 25% risk of inheriting a "double dose" of **r** genes which may cause a serious birth defect
2. a 25% chance of inheriting two **N**s, thus being unaffected
3. a 50% chance of being a carrier as both parents are

Source: Modified from "Genetic Counseling," a booklet prepared by The March of Dimes Birth Defect Foundation, pp. 14 and 15.

screening program and routine selective abortion, we *could* practically eliminate some genetic disorders. By detecting and destroying all affected and carrier fetuses, the deleterious gene would not be passed on to future generations. A more extreme measure could be an intensive genetic screening program to detect all future parents who are carriers of genetic disorders. Laws *could* be enacted to prevent them from marrying, or to require that they be identified in the population, or to have all their fetuses submitted to nonvoluntary prenatal screening. You may be surprised to discover that all these possibilities have been discussed at least, and some have become law or routine practice in some jurisdictions. From this broad sketch of key developments and crucial areas that require deliberation, let us turn to some issues in more detail.

GENETIC TESTING AND NEW KINDS OF DECISIONS

STATE HEALTH DEPARTMENTS HAVE A LIST OF REPORTABLE DISEASES. PHYSICIANS ARE required to report to the health department cases of tuberculosis, venereal diseases, and other communicable illnesses. Similarly, law enforcement agencies require physicians to report suicides, violent injuries, and unexplained deaths. *Now, imagine that sometime in the future . . .*

Dr. Lu has just developed a test for a genetic disease frequently associated with antisocial behavior. The carrier state for this disease can be assayed in a blood test of potential parents.

The health department is considering the possibility of making this test a requirement for obtaining a marriage license, just as it now requires a test for veneral disease.

Some Questions to Consider
1. Would you support this requirement?
2. Is the society obligated to set up such programs to eliminate the possibility of passing on genetic disorders?
3. What would be the impact of such testing on the privacy of childbearing decisions made by parents?

Genetic tests yield information about individuals. They indicate whether a person is a carrier of a disease. In the future, they may indicate even more subtle traits, such as a predisposition for cancer or personality type. Prenatal tests provide information about an unborn fetus, including its sex, whether it is affected by certain genetic disorders.

If the results of genetic tests indicate that a potential parent couple both carry recessive genes for a particular disease, then they know the familiar odds: a one-in-four chance of producing a child not affected or a carrier, a two-in-four chance of producing a child who is a carrier, a one-in-four chance of producing a child who is affected. Personally, the couple faces several tough choices not faced by previous generations of parents. *Knowing* they are carriers, should they try to have children? If there is a pregnancy, should they have prenatal screening performed? If the fetus is affected or a carrier, should they have it aborted?

In the realm of public policy, we all face the following sorts of choices. With the capacity to detect carriers and affected fetuses, should there be mandatory screening programs? Should parents of fetuses known to be affected be influenced, for example through a tax-incentive program that would reward parents for not having affected children? Should use of genetic testing, prenatal testing, and genetic screening be used extensively by a society to reduce the number of births of affected fetuses or to eliminate some genetic diseases, or should all such programs be voluntary? Genetic testing, screening, and prenatal testing provide genetic information about adults, newborns, and fetuses. Through required public health programs and selective abortion, many inherited disorders could be reduced and perhaps virtually eliminated. (Spontaneous mutation might cause, however, a rare recurrence.)

Mrs. Whipple loved her second son, the simple-minded one, better than she loved the other two children put together. . . . He seemed to be accusing her of something. Maybe He remembered that time she boxed His ears, maybe He had been scared that day with the bull, maybe He had slept cold and couldn't tell her about it. Maybe He knew they were sending Him away for good and all because they were too poor to keep Him. Whatever it was, Mrs. Whipple couldn't bear to think of it. She began to cry, frightfully, and wrapped her arms tight around Him. His head rolled on her shoulder: she had loved Him as much as she possibly could, there were Adna and Emly who had to be thought of too, there was nothing she could do to make up to Him for His life. Oh, what a mortal pity He was ever born.

—Katherine Ann Porter,
"He"

There is a long-standing precedent for required public health programs. Public health laws that require vaccinations, for example, need compliance with medical directives not only for the benefit of the individual, but also for the welfare of other citizens who would be protected from contracting a contagious disease. Some commentators argue that the same moral and legal justification applies to requiring mandatory public health laws that would reduce or eliminate genetic diseases. Joseph Fletcher is one. Excerpts from his utilitarian moral argument are at the end of this chapter. Others argue that the privacy of childbearing decisions must be upheld. A report from the Hastings Center makes this argument. It, too, is at the conclusion of this chapter.

An alternative to nonvoluntary screening programs is the voluntary education and screening programs established by individual organizations. For example, Tay Sachs disease is a genetic disorder especially prevalent among Ashkenazic Jews. In the United States, Jewish organizations and synagogues have created in recent years special education programs with voluntary genetic testing and counseling. Other groups knowing of specific genetic disorders prevalent in their ethnic heritage have established similar programs. In some situations where there is strong opposition to abortion, for example among the Greek Orthodox, information gained from genetic testing of parents or prenatal testing of fetuses may or may not influence choice of spouse, and only rarely would lead to a decision to abort an affected fetus. Instead, such information might help parents prepare emotionally and financially for having a child affected by a genetic disorder. What individual groups do on a voluntary basis may provide an alternative use of genetic testing technologies to government-sponsored mass screening programs.

There is an important public policy decision we must make—one which follows from our earlier discussions in chapters 2, 6, and 7. It has to do with the *allocation* of genetic and prenatal testing. Short of mandatory, universal screening programs, there are decisions to be made about who should have what degree of access to such medical tests. Generally, those who argue *for access* to abortion and the maximum freedom of choice for the woman favor wide distribution of genetic testing; those *opposed* to abortion generally want to limit it. Should government funds or private third-party payers, like insurance companies, pay for genetic testing? While many middle-class and wealthy women know about genetic testing and have used it, many other women do not know about the kind of information it can provide or about its availability. Should government funds be used to educate all women and to increase accessibility to genetic testing? Once again, the allocation question we discussed in chapter 7 emerges: should education, income, and other class factors determine the degree of access to health care?

MORE INFORMATION, FURTHER CHOICES

In addition to the new kinds of parenting decisions put to potential parents and society by the development of genetic testing, screening, and prenatal testing in the 1960s and 1970s, there are further questions about how such genetic information ought to be managed.

The prospect of nefarious application is *not* what makes genetic knowledge unique. Rather, its uniqueness lies in the manner in which "knowing" the genetics of something changes it.

For example, the simple act of acquiring prenatal genetic information about a fetus—whether or not he is carrying a particular gene, or if he will develop a genetically determined disease later in his life—automatically sets into motion a train of events which themselves change that individual's future. At the very moment you acquire a "bit" of genetic information about a fetus (or any person, for that matter), you have begun to define him in entirely novel

terms. You tell him (and sometimes others) something about where he came from and who is responsible for what he is now. You project who he may or may not become in the future. You set certain limits on his potential. You say something about what his children will be like, and whether or not he will be encouraged or discouraged to think of himself as a parent. In this way the information you obtain changes both the individual who possesses it, and in turn the future of that information itself.[1]

—Marc Lappé,
Chief, Office of Health, Law and Value,
California Department of Health

AGAIN, IMAGINE A POSSIBLE FUTURE SITUATION. YOUR FATHER, NOW 43 YEARS OLD, STARTED to become forgetful, untidy, and showed some involuntary jerking motions in his arms and legs. You encouraged him to go to the doctor, who diagnosed Huntington's Chorea. In discussing the problem with your father's physician this morning, you learned that Huntington's Chorea is a genetically determined disease and that it follows a course of progressive dementia, causes abnormal movements, and slowly leads to death. The term "genetically determined" stuck in your mind, and finally you asked. You have a fifty-fifty chance of developing the disease yourself. There is no cure and no treatment.

Realizing your concern, the physician explained to you that he could send you for some newly developed tests to determine whether you too have the disease and will develop symptoms in later years.

Some Questions to Consider
1. Do you want genetic testing for yourself or for your children?
2. Do you have any obligations to future generations to decrease the frequency of a genetically determined disease such as Huntington's Chorea?
3. Whom would you want and whom would you *not* want to know that you had a heritable disease? Your spouse? Employer? Insurance company? A government health agency?

How shall we manage information gained from genetic testing and screening? This question is crucial for several reasons:

1. Symptoms may not manifest themselves for many years, even decades, in the life of the person known to be affected.
2. Diagnosis now is extended into prediction, with fair accuracy, of direct genetic disorders or even genetically caused propensities for future diseases.

1. Marc Lappé, "Moral Obligations, and the Fallacies of Genetic Control," *Theological Studies* 33 (September 1972): 412.

3. Genetic counselors have discovered that genetic information can raise emotionally devastating questions about self-worth, desirability as a parent or future parent, or profound existential questions about one's fate and faith.
4. Others may have genetic information—other family members, insurance companies, the government—and make decisions that influence a person's life with or without his or her knowledge.
5. Genetic information can be misinterpreted dangerously.
6. Genetic tests are not without error.

As of now, we lack clear-cut policies and guidelines for determining how genetic information ought to be stored or conveyed. The medical technology of genetic testing and screening has outrun any hammered-out or emergent consensus on how to manage it. It has pushed medical diagnosis into a wholly new realm. As we saw in chapter 5, there are serious arguments for providing full medical information to patients, but there are equally serious arguments against full disclosure. Genetic testing may someday indicate that a newborn will, at the age of forty, manifest symptoms of a disease for which there is no known cure. Should, and at what age, this child be *told* this kind of information? Should it be withheld by the doctor from the parents? Must society limit access to such information by the government, schools, employers, insurance companies, or others who may make decisions that affect a person's opportunities in life?

Although genetic testing yields highly reliable information, it is not one-hundred-percent accurate. In the case of testing fetuses, a *false negative* result (indicating there is no genetic disorder when in fact there is) or a *false positive* result (indicating there is a genetic disorder when there is not) can lead to parents' making decisions about abortion on the basis of inaccurate information.

Genetic information can be misinterpreted. Consider the misunderstanding of the function of an extra Y chromosome several years ago. A mass murderer, Richard Speck, was an XYY type. This discovery and its surrounding publicity, coupled with the ideas of some leading geneticists, caused, in the 1960s, at least two states to perform genetic screening on boys in juvenile homes to detect and identify XYY types. Subsequently, it has been discovered that a simplistic connection between an extra Y chromosome and aggressive behavior cannot be made. Similarly, in the 1960s and 1970s there was confusion about sickle-cell trait among American blacks. Although an asset in tropical climates, in temperate climates sickle-cell anemia is a debilitating and tragic disease for those affected. In the last two decades, programs to screen American blacks have been run by employers, insurance companies, and military academies; carriers of sickle-cell trait were detected and eliminated from employment, military service, or insurance coverage because it was believed they were affected, even if they showed no symptoms at all and were, in fact, in no way affected by anemia. If it were not for genetic testing, *only* those black children who are affected would be known, because the symptoms would be manifest; before the development of genetic testing, carriers were undetected for sickle-cell, just as for all other genetic disorders.

Information gained from genetic testing is potent. Inaccurate information or misunderstood information can lead to adverse decisions that have real impact on the lives of individuals. Because this information may be known outside the patient-doctor relationship there is a strong possibility of mismanagement. At least one famous court case exonerated an employer from the responsibility to provide an employee with information gained from the employer's health-screening program. In *Lotspeich v. Chance Vought Aircraft Corporation*,[2] the employer was not held accountable for having withheld information from one of its employees that she had tuberculosis, which had been detected in a routine testing program. She showed no symptoms as of then, and she was not told. Because the information was not gained within a conventional doctor-patient relationship, the customary rules of informed consent and confidentiality did not apply, the court ruled.

GENETIC ENGINEERING AND NEW RISKS

Of all the developments in applied genetics, the most challenging in its potential ramifications for our self-image and evolution as a species is genetic engineering. A series of significant discoveries by molecular biologists over the last fifteen years has culminated in the technologies of genetic engineering. The discovery of restrictive enzymes in the early 1970s enabled the actual slicing and recombining of the long strands of DNA. Because genes "instruct" the cell or organism, the recombined DNA causes subsequent development of the cell or organism to be altered. For example, the DNA in a laboratory strain of *Escherichia coli*, derived from the common colon bacillus normally found in the human intestinal tract, can be "cut" with restriction enzymes, and DNA from another organism can then be spliced into it. Perhaps genetic material that "instructs" the production of insulin might be inserted. Therapeutic benefits of this sort of procedure are envisioned, for diabetics in this example, and further advances eventually may include gene therapy, which would replace defective genes with normal genes.

In early 1980, there was a controversial attempt by American medical personnel to replace defective hemoglobin genes in the bone marrow of patients in Italy and Israel. The experiments were done there because the Institutional Review Board (IRB) of the researchers' home institution, the

2. *Lotspeich v. Chance Vought Aircraft Corporation*, 369 S.W.2d 705 (Tex. Civ. App., 1963).

University of California at Los Angeles, wanted them to do more animal experiments before experimenting on humans. The researchers replied that experimental attempts at gene therapy were the only hope for patients with fatal disorders like beta thalassemia, a severe anemia arising from an inherited hemoglobin abnormality.

NOW THINK ABOUT A CASE IN WHICH GENETIC ENGINEERING ENTERS AS A POSSIBILITY. YOUR one-year-old son has just been diagnosed as having beta thalassemia. Your doctor explains to you that this disease will cause your son to be chronically anemic, will delay his growth and development, will cause some abnormalities of his skeleton, will require him to receive multiple transfusions, and probably will result in his death as he reaches young adulthood.

Your doctor goes on to explain that there is now an experimental technique for correcting this genetic abnormality. It would involve removing some bone marrow from your son and altering it genetically. Any bone marrow remaining in his body would be destroyed through irradiation and medication. After that, the genetically altered marrow would be reinjected in the hope that it would repopulate his bone marrow with normal, hemoglobin-producing cells. If the technique proved successful, your son would enjoy a normal life. The doctor is candid in telling you that the reintroduced bone marrow might not take and that there is a risk of increasing the possibility that your son would develop a malignancy later because of the radiation and drugs.

Some Questions to Consider
1. Would you authorize the experimental technique?
2. How would you weigh the personal benefits versus risks?
3. Would you feel any obligation to contribute to the advancement of biomedical science by allowing this kind of experiment because it is necessary for the successful development of medical technology?

Genetic experimentation carries a possible hazard to public health and safety. The presumed danger is in the release of genetically altered organisms into the environment, where their behavior would be unpredictable. Such concerns reached a peak in early 1975, when an international conference of scientists, attorneys, and others interested in the effects of genetic experimentation was called at Asilomar, California. Working with representatives from the National Institutes of Health, the members of the conference developed guidelines, which were promulgated by NIH in 1976, requiring that all federally funded research in genetics be undertaken in "stage-three" laboratory conditions (the same restrictions imposed on the most dangerous kind of laboratory work, with bacteria). Voluntary compliance was given by private laboratories. By the early 1980s, these guidelines had been substantially relaxed, although most genetic research is still conducted very carefully. The significance of these developments is that for the first time in history, a group of scientists initiated a moratorium on their research, helped create research guidelines, and complied officially and voluntarily.

Ongoing developments in genetic engineering may render inadequate our current regulations regarding experimentation on human subjects and threats to public health. For example, new microbes created by genetic engineering may have exotic new capabilities. Some scientists like to mention the development of oil-"eating" microbes that could be released into oil spills in the ocean. A neat way of cleaning up an oil slick, but any such experiment would involve a significant risk. Through nature's own "genetic engineering," which has been going on since long before humankind began doing it, unknown mutations with unforeseen qualities might develop. In addition to this kind of an intentional release of new microbe into the environment, there are unknown risks due to accidental release. Also, as we learned in 1945, there is always the possibility that technological innovations can be beaten into swords. The prospects of biowarfare are awesome and frightening, but must be confronted.

Genetic engineering is a powerful new medical technology. Its actual accomplishments so far are primitive, compared with expected developments. Because it manipulates the most fundamental elements of organic life, genes, in much the same way that nuclear physicists manipulate atoms, serious and legitimate concerns have been raised about present and future developments. Clearly there are risks. Experimentation on human beings is a necessary phase in the successful development of any new medical technology. A few individuals and families will face the dilemma of deciding whether to take the risk. The society at large has produced rules, in the form of federal guidelines, for experimentation on human subjects. Researchers, citizens, legislators, members of IRBs, and others will be confronted with decisions regarding genetic research and experimentation. What risks connected with genetic engineering are we willing to accept? How can we responsibly control such necessary and inevitable risks?

One egg, one embryo, one adult—normality. But a bokanovskified egg will bud, will proliferate, will divide. From eight to ninety-six buds, and every bud will grow into a perfectly formed embryo, and every embryo into a full-sized adult. Making ninety-six human beings grow where only one grew before. Progress.

—Aldous Huxley,
Brave New World

GENETICS AND OUR FUTURE

Through existing and future applied genetic technologies, the evolution of the human species and our environment can be influenced intentionally or accidentally. The history of eugenics and its murderous turn under Hitler raise legitimate questions about the purpose for which applied genetics might be used. Growing knowledge about how vulnerable the environment is to humankind's technological innovations and about environmental threats to human health raise similar questions. The failures and mixed results that have characterized our past moral preparation for technological developments make many people dubious about our capacity to direct responsibly the evolution of organic life, especially the future of the human species. Assuming that genetic technologies will increase our power to influence evolution, we could speculate that future developments will be haphazard and accompanied by unforeseen consequences. To be effective, an intentional effort to control evolution would necessarily have to be *international.* Our record with international control of nuclear warfare, for example, does not inspire confidence that even the most serious of problems are approached responsibly and reasonably in our current international behavior.

Based on these precedents, some have argued that we ought to slow down genetic research. Others argue that pure scientific inquiry cannot be fettered. Sometimes the practical argument is advanced that if "we" do not keep ahead in such areas as applied genetics, "they" will. What has become a classic modern dilemma emerges in applied genetics, too: the unrestricted quest for knowledge *versus* concerns about its applications, misapplications, and unintended results. This dilemma shows up clearly in the debate over the level of government investment in genetic research and the arrangements for private financing, especially when the primary motive for investment is profit.

The possibilities of genetic engineering and evolutionary control illustrate the fundamental dilemmas raised by the new capabilities conferred by scientific knowledge. Society has entered an age of intervention, in which the automatic operation of natural processes is increasingly, through informed intervention, brought consciously into the orbit of human purpose. Many events that humanity formerly could regard only as a boon or a scourge—an act of God or of nature—are now the partial product of human decision and intervention. If human beings do not have the capability today to invent new organisms or to initiate life itself, they may soon have that capability. If they cannot today consciously and fully control the behavior of large ecosystems, that power is not far

beyond what has already been achieved. The humility of individuals understandably shrinks from awesome powers that were earlier assigned to divine will. It was not, however, the humility of individuals that conferred these emerging capabilities or is called on to control them today. It was the social interaction of individuals, operating through social institutions, that brought us to the present fateful decision making. Imperfect though they are, our social institutions built the platform for the age of intervention.[3]

—Clifford Grobstein,
Department of Science, Technology and Public Affairs,
University of California, San Diego

ARE WE PREPARED?

Developments in genetics incorporate and in some ways raise to a higher level of importance and urgency many of the issues discussed in previous chapters in this book.

- The questions "When does human life begin?" and "What is a person?"—as analyzed in chapter 2—may now be joined by "What is a human being?"
- Information yielded by genetic testing presents new childbearing decisions to parents or would-be parents.
- Genetic information may predict the development of disease that will occur much later in a person's life; new strains are placed on the conventional doctor-patient relationship in the management of this information.
- In an age of computer-stored genetic information, key questions are raised about confidentiality.
- It seems that current attempts to define and to practice the ideals of informed consent and self-determination may become even more nebulous and threatened.
- The distribution of benefits and risks raises an awkward and uncomfortable question: Will the economically advantaged (and insured) receive the benefits of genetic developments while the poor take the risks?
- What shall be the moral *purpose* of new medical technologies, such as those emerging in applied genetics?

These are some of the areas in which individuals and the society at large will be required to make vital choices, *beginning now*. The benefits of modern medical developments are clear: now, from time to time, the

3. Clifford Grobstein, "The Recombinant-DNA Debate," *Scientific American*, July 1977, p. 32.

unintended side effects are *becoming* equally clear. Our best hope in a future filled with such vital choices is to be *prepared* for what is ahead.

In the course of these few pages, we have attempted to outline the shape of the moral and public policy decisions created by modern medical developments. Throughout the book, and especially in this last chapter, we have tried to indicate those areas in which the most important and pressing questions will arise. The best way to go into the unknowable future is with informed opinions about the present and knowledgeable speculation about that which the future may hold. It is your best hope individually and the best hope of all of us collectively.

SELECTED READINGS
Protecting Privacy in a Genetic Screening Program[4]

Since screening programs acquire genetic information from large numbers of normal and asymptomatic (e.g., carrier state) individuals and families, often after only brief medical contact, their operation generally falls outside the usual patient-initiated doctor-patient relation. As a result, traditional applications of ethical guidelines for confidentiality and individual physician responsibility are uncertain in mass screening programs. Thus, we believe it important that attempts be made now to clarify some ethical, social and legal questions concerning the establishment and operation of such programs. . . .

It is crucial that screening programs be structured on the basis of one or more clearly identified goals and that such goals be formulated well before screening actually begins. . . . [W]e believe the most important goals are those that either contribute to improving the health of persons who suffer from genetic disorders, or allow carriers for a given variant gene to make informed choices regarding reproduction, or move toward alleviating the anxieties of families and communities faced with the prospect of serious genetic disease. The following are representative statements of goals that have been used to justify screening programs.

Such benefits may arise from enabling couples found by screening to be at risk for transmitting a genetic disease to take genetic information into account in making responsible decisions about having or not having children. . . .

Laboratory research and theoretical studies have had a major role in helping to understand fundamental aspects of human genetic diseases. In addition, however, some large-scale screening programs may be needed to determine frequencies of rare diseases and to establish new correlations between genes or groups of genes and disease. . . .

Although little is known about the possible beneficial (or detrimental) effects of most deleterious recessive genes in the heterozygous state, the reduction of their

4. Excerpts from the Hasting Center's Institute of Society, Ethics and the Life Sciences, Research Group on Ethical, Social and Legal Issues in Genetic Counseling and Genetic Engineering, "Ethical and Social Issues in Screening for Genetic Disease," excerpted by permission of the *New England Journal of Medicine* 286 (1972): 1129–32.

frequency would be one way to decrease the occurrence of suffering caused by their homozygous manifestations. Nevertheless, as a goal of screening programs, the means required to approach this objective appear to be both practically and morally unacceptable. Virtually everyone carries a small number of deleterious or lethal recessive genes, and to reduce the frequency of a particular recessive gene to near the level maintained by recurrent mutation, most or all persons heterozygous for that gene would have either to refrain from procreation entirely or to monitor all their offspring in utero and abort not only affected homozygote fetuses but also the larger number of heterozygote carriers for the gene. . . .

As a general principle, we strongly urge that no screening program have policies that would in any way impose constraints on childbearing by individuals of any specific genetic constitution, or would stigmatize couples who, with full knowledge of the genetic risks, still desire children of their own. It is unjustifiable to promulgate standards for normalcy based on genetic constitution. Consequently, genetic screening programs should be conducted on a voluntary basis. Although vaccination against contagious diseases and premarital blood tests are sometimes made mandatory to protect the public health, there is currently no public-health justification for mandatory screening for the prevention of genetic disease. The conditions being tested for in screening programs are neither "contagious" nor, for the most part, susceptible to treatment at present.

Screening should be conducted only with the informed consent of those tested or of the parents or legal representatives of minors. We seriously question the rationale of screening preschool minors or preadolescents for sickle-cell disease or trait since there is a substantial danger of stigmatization and little medical value in detecting the carrier state at this age. . . .

Since genetic screening is generally undertaken with relatively untried testing procedures and is vitally concerned with the acquisition of new knowledge, it ought properly to be considered a form of "human experimentation." Although most screening entails only minimum physical hazard for the participants, there is a risk of possible psychologic or social injury, and screening programs should consequently be conducted according to the guidelines set forth by HEW for the protection of research subjects.

A screening program should fully and clearly disclose to the community and all persons being screened its policies for informing those screened of the results of the tests performed on them. As a general rule all unambiguous diagnostic results should be made available to the person, his legal representative, or a physician authorized by him. Where full disclosure is not practiced, the burden of justifying nondisclosure lies with those who would withhold information. . . .

Well-trained genetic counselors should be readily available to provide adequate assistance (including repeated counseling sessions if necessary) for persons identified as heterozygotes or more rarely homozygotes by the screening program. As a general rule, counseling should be nondirective, with an emphasis on informing the client and not making decisions for him. . . .

As part of the educational process that precedes the actual testing program, the nature and cost of available therapies or maintenance programs for affected offspring, combined with an understandable description of their possible benefits and risks, should be given to all persons to be screened. . . .

Even if the above guidelines are followed, some risk will remain that the information derived from genetic screening will be misused. Such misuse or misinterpretation must be seen as one of the principal potentially deleterious consequences of screening programs. . . . In view of such collateral risks of screening, it is essential that each program's periodic review include careful consideration of the social and psychologic ramifications of its operation.

Protecting the Quality of Life[5]

An editorial by Dr. Malcolm Watts in the journal of the California Medical Association in 1970 remarked that "man exercises ever more certain and effective control" over the quality of human life. "It will become necessary and acceptable to place relative rather than absolute values on such things as human lives, the use of scarce resources, and the various elements which are to make up the quality of life or of living which is to be sought."[a] All of this, he said, requires "a new ethic" in "a rational development" of "what is almost certain to be a biologically oriented world society."

Physicians in the past, the editorial points out, have tried "to preserve, protect, repair, prolong, and enhance every human life which comes under their surveillance." This was the old vitalistic, undiscriminating sanctity-or-quantity-of-life ethics, now giving way to a responsible, decisional quality-of-life ethics. To repair and prolong lives, indiscriminately, may be a kind of technical virtuosity but it is not *control*. To control means to choose, and therefore any absolute morality about always keeping life going, before or after birth, regardless of quality considerations, is the very opposite of control and a denial of quality.

If we choose family size we should choose family health. This is what the controls of reproductive medicine make possible. Public health and sanitation have greatly reduced human ills; now the major ills have become genetic and congenital. They can be reduced by medical controls. We ought to protect our families from the emotional and material burden of such diseased individuals, and from the misery of their simply "existing" (not *living*) in a nearby "warehouse" or public institution. . . .

If the State is morally justified in repelling an unwelcome invader, why should not a woman do so when burdened or invaded by an unwelcome pregnancy? And why shouldn't the family be protected from an idiot or terribly diseased sibling? Control is human and rational; submission, the opposite of control, is subhuman. Suffering and misfortune cannot be utterly escaped, it is true, and human beings can grow tremendously in pain and disappointment. But a basic ethical principle of medicine and health care is nonetheless the minimization of human suffering, by deliberate control.

5. Excerpts from Joseph Fletcher, *The Ethics of Genetic Control* (Garden City, N.Y.: Doubleday, Anchor, 1974), pp. 156–57, 157–58, 181–83.

a. "A New Ethic for Medicine and Society," *California Medicine* 113 (September 1970): 67–68.

Producing our children by "sexual roulette" without preconceptive and uterine control, simply taking "pot luck" from random sexual combinations, is irresponsible—now that we can be genetically selective and know how to monitor against congenital infirmities. As we learn to direct mutations medically we should do so. Not to control when we can is immoral. This way it will be much easier to assure our children that they really are here because they were *wanted*, that they were born "on purpose."

Controlling the quality of life is not negative; it just rejects what fails to come up to a positive standard. The new biology equips us to save and improve the defective, as well as to maintain a sensible standard. . . .

A good illustration of the tension between rights and regulation takes shape in trying to control hereditary disease. Each of us carries from five to ten genetic faults. If they match up in sexual roulette, tragedy results. How can we avoid or curtail the danger? Denmark prohibits marriages of certain couples unless they are sterilized. But if this method of control and prevention is used, or any other, how do we find out *who* are the ones who should not marry or, if they do, should not have babies by the natural or coital mode? Screening by one means or another is the obvious way to fulfill our obligation to potential children, as well as to the community which has to suffer when defectives are born.

The law in most countries is far behind our emerging medical information. People are not required to make their bad genes known to their mates nor are physicians required to reveal the facts. A man with polycystic kidney disease is not required to let it be known—even though it is highly immoral (unjust) to keep knowledge of such a hereditary disaster (renal failure in middle age) from his children and those they marry. Medical genetics will continue to isolate more and more such diseases, so that as our ability to prevent disease and tragedy increases so does the moral guilt of secrecy, indifference to the consequences for others, and fatalistic inaction.

Conquering infectious diseases reduces the cause of the trouble, but to conquer genetic diseases *increases* the cause or source of the trouble. This dysgenic effect is the first big-scale moral dilemma for medicine—truly a dilemma. Infections come from the environment around us but genetic faults come from within us, and therefore any line of genetic sufferers allowed to propagate will spread their disease through more and more carriers. As we cut down on the infectious diseases we are threatened with a relative rise in deaths and debility due to genetic disorders. We are now approaching a situation in which genetic causes account for as many *or more* deaths than "disease" in the popular sense.

Our moral obligation to undergo voluntary screening, if it is indicated, is too obvious to underline. The squeeze here, ethically, is that the social good often requires *mass* screening. When it is voluntary it is "nicer," as we see in the popular acceptance of tests for cervical cancer. But let it be compulsory if need be, for the common good—Hardin's "mutual coercion mutually agreed upon." Francis Crick has said that "if we can get across to people the idea that their children are not entirely their own business and that it is not a private matter, it would be an enormous step forward." The biophysicist Leroy Augenstein estimated in 1972 that a total of 6 per cent of births or one out of seventeen, are defective. Of these, he said, forty thousand to fifty thousand children every year "are so defective that they don't know that they are human beings."[b] His figures are more impressive than his formulation, however; if an individual cannot "know" he is a human being he is not a human being.

Parents of adopted children and donors of AID [Artificial Insemination by Donor] are much more carefully screened and selected than "natural" parents—which is logically ridiculous even though we can understand how it came about. A socially conscientious system would be a national registry; blood and skin tests done routinely at birth and fed into a computer-gene scanner would pick up all anomalies, and they would be printed out on data cards and filed; then when marriage licenses are applied for, the cards would be read in comparison machines to find incompatibilities and homozygous conditions.

The objection is, predictably, that it would "violate" a "right"—the right to privacy. It is even said, in a brazen attack on reason itself, that we have a "right to *not* know." Which is more important, the alleged "privacy" or the good of the couple as well as of their progeny and society? (The couple could unite anyway, of course, but on the condition Denmark makes—that sterilization is done for one or both of them. And they could even still have children by medical and donor assistance, bypassing their own faulty fertility.)

Screening is no more an invasion of privacy than "contact tracing" in the treatment of venereal disease, or income tax and public health records, or compulsory fluoridation of the water, or the age-old codes of consanguinity (which were only based on nonsense). A good education for those who balk would be a week's stay in the wards of a state institution for the "retarded"—a term used to cover a host of terrible distortions of humanity. Just let them *see* the nature and extent of it; that would convince them.

ANNOTATED BIBLIOGRAPHY
Books and Articles

Lappé, Marc. *Genetic Politics: The Limits of Biological Control.* New York: Simon and Schuster, 1979. A popular, well-written work on multiple moral and public policy problems in applied genetics.

Omenn, Gilbert S. "Genetics and Epidemiology: Medical Interventions and Public Policy." *Social Biology* 26 (Summer 1979): 117–25. A physician and policy expert writes on the connections between medicine and public policy.

Powledge, Tabitha M., and John Fletcher. "Guidelines for the Ethical, Social, and Legal Issues in Prenatal Diagnosis." *New England Journal of Medicine* 300 (January 1979): 168–72. This readable essay is a Hastings Center Task Force Report that has been widely disseminated and widely quoted.

Wade, Nicholas. *The Ultimate Experiment: Man-Made Evolution.* New York: Walker, 1977. A science writer presents a vivid depiction of contemporary problems and options.

b. "Birth Defects," in *Humanistic Perspectives in Medical Ethics,* ed. M. Visscher (London: Pemberton Publishing Co., 1972), p. 207.

Anthologies

Gastel, Barbara, et al. *Maternal Serum Alpha-Fetoprotein: Issues in the Prenatal Screening and Diagnosis of Neural Tube Defects.* Washington, D.C.: Government Printing Office, 1981. A recent symposium on genetic screening that explores ethical, legal, and social options and problems.

Jackson, David A., and Stephen P. Stich, eds. *The Recombinant DNA Debate.* Englewood Cliffs, N.J.: Prentice-Hall, 1979. A difficult but well-constructed essay on problems of molecular genetic research involving the recombining of genes (so-called gene splicing).

Lappé, Marc, and Robert S. Morrison, eds. "Ethical and Scientific Issues Posed by Human Uses of Molecular Genetics." *Annals of the New York Academy of Sciences* 265 (1976): 1–208. A special issue that includes several important essays.

Milunsky, Aubrey, ed. *Genetic Disorders and the Fetus.* New York: Plenum Press, 1979. A very thorough medical, moral, and policy exploration.

Articles from the *Encyclopedia of Bioethics*

Genetic Aspects of Human Behavior
 I. State of the Art *Irving I. Gottesman*
 II. Males with Sex Chromosome Abnormalities (XYY and XXY Genotypes) *Ernest B. Hook*
 III. Race Differences in Intelligence *John C. Loehlin*
 IV. Genetics and Mental Disorders *Irving I. Gottesman*
 V. Philosophical and Ethical Issues *Arthur L. Caplan*
Genetic Constitution and Environmental Conditioning *René Dubos*
Genetic Diagnosis and Counseling
 I. Genetic Diagnosis *Robert F. Murray, Jr.*
 II. Genetic Counseling *Robert F. Murray, Jr.*
Genetic Screening *Tabitha M. Powledge*
Genetics and the Law *Margery W. Shaw*
Prenatal Diagnosis
 I. Clinical Aspects *Aubrey Milunsky*
 II. Ethical Issues *John C. Fletcher*

Literature

Huxley, Aldous. *Brave New World.* 1932. New York: Bantam, 1958. "Pregnancy and Childbirth" is an archaic topic for the people of the year 632 After Ford who are growing bottled babies in identical sets. Startling in 1932 for its vision of the future, uncanny in the 1980s for its accuracy, *Brave New World* explores the impact on human values of the capacity of biomedical science to alter the means and results of human reproduction.

Audio/Visual

"The Gene Engineers." "NOVA" series, 57-minute film or videotape. Sale or rental, Time/Life Video, Eisenhower Drive, Paramus, N.J., 07652. The scientific, moral, and legal questions surrounding genetic engineering are raised—both the prospective benefits and possible dangers.

INDEX

This book is one of four publications intended to engage a broad range of persons in informed decision-making regarding key health and human value questions. Each publication has a usefulness of its own, while all four comprise a convenient series.

The main text, *Health and Human Values: A Guide to Making Your Own Decisions*, contains case studies and background discussions of important moral, medical, and legal topics, selected readings from prominent writers in medicine, theology, philosophy, law, and related fields, and annotated bibliographies of recommended articles, books, anthologies, literary works, and audio-visual resources.

Also available in the series are:

• *Leader's Manual* for *Health and Human Values: A Guide to Making Your Own Decisions*. For persons leading study groups, continuing professional education courses, and academic classes concentrating on biomedical-ethical issues, this manual offers suggestions for making best use of the cases and discussions in the primary study book, organizing learning activities, and selecting further references for group discussion.

• *Biomedical-Ethical Issues: A Digest of Law and Policy Development*. This handbook contains excerpts and summaries of influential court decisions, state and federal legislation, and federal guidelines, as well as policy statements from various religious and professional organizations, related to biomedical-ethical issues. By providing excerpts, the digest enables the general reader and the legal specialist to understand the recent evolution of public policy and to recognize those areas of public policy that remain incomplete and, in some cases, contradictory.

• *Human Values in Medicine and Health Care: Audio-Visual Resources*. Approximately 400 audio-visual items are listed; most are annotated, and all include full information about purchase and rental costs and the names and addresses of distributors. Two indexes list the items by topic and by format (film, videocassette, audio-cassette, or slide/tape).

These publications are offered to the general reader, patients and their families, physicians, nurses, and other health care practitioners, clergy, attorneys, educators, students, legislators, and activists who seek to influence public policy. It is hoped that they will be used to help inform our thinking about the crucial health and human value choices facing us all.

ORDERING INFORMATION

To place an order for any book in the Health and Human Values series, write or call:

Yale University Press
Sales Department
92A Yale Station
New Haven, CT 06520

Tel.: 203 432-4840